Lifegain

LIFEGAIN

The exciting new program
that will change your
health–and your life

Robert F. Allen, Ph.D.

with SHIRLEY LINDE

HUMAN RESOURCES INSTITUTE / Morristown, N.J.

Copyright © 1981 by Robert F. Allen.

83 84 85 / 10 9 8 7 6 5 4 3 2 1

Library of Congress Cataloging in Publication Data

Allen, Robert Francis, 1928-
   Lifegain: the exciting new program that will
change your health — and your life.

   Bibliography.
   1. Health. 2. Health behavior. I. Linde,
Shirley Motter, joint author. II. Title.
RA776.A377   613   80-25991
ISBN 0-8385-5671-X

Text design: Judith F. Warm
Cover design: Lawrence Daniels & Friends, Inc.

PRINTED IN THE UNITED STATES OF AMERICA

Contents

Preface

How healthy are you?

Is health just not being sick? Or is it more than that: having energy to burn at the end of the day, feeling super great, happy, satisfied with what you've done, looking forward to a long and healthy future, feeling good about yourself and others?

Most of us are born with the potential to feel more than just "not sick." But something happens along the way. That something is our culture, our antihealth culture, that often, without our being aware of it, controls the way we live. It encourages us to be overweight, underexercised, improperly nourished, tense, accident prone, and unfit.

If you're like most of us, you've already tried to change. If you were not concerned, if you really didn't want to do anything about your health, you would probably not be reading this book.

If you've lost the same pounds many times, or tried to give up smoking, or swore you'd have more fun, or tried to improve your life in some other way — and failed — it is probably because of your lifestyle and your inability to get your culture to support you. Lifegain shows you a way to harness your own power and the power of culture, and then put them to work in your life and in the lives of those around you.

Lifegain is a new system, based on 25 years of research, that is helping people across the country decide for themselves just how healthy they can be. It is a system for gaining control of your health by understanding yourself and the culture that influences you and by changing both when necessary.

We hope that this approach will mean as much to you as it has to us and to the others who have entered the Lifegain program.

1

A New and Exciting Approach to Health

OUR CULTURES ARE KILLING US

The village well was poisoned and people fell sick. The doctors, the nurses, the villagers all ran about buying new beds, giving medicines, providing life-long care for those permanently crippled or diseased. They became very adept at treating the ill. They refined the medicines, discovered new and stronger antidotes, trained people to care for the sick, built beautiful build-ings to accommodate the chronically ill. Better treatment procedures were invented with marvelous mechanical devices; emergency services were de-veloped to a remarkable degree of efficiency; there never had been better medical care anywhere. But the patients kept coming and the statistics kept rising, for no one treated the source of the problem—the poisoned well.

Our cultures are poisoned wells today. They do not encourage people to be healthy. Even our medical care system is not a health-promoting one; it's a curative system that focuses on our illness after the damage has been done.

We practice patch-up medicine. We spend billions for surgery, for coronary care units, for kidney dialysis machines, for radiation therapy and chemical treatment for cancer.

Our efforts and our money go to treat the results of our illness culture.

Researchers produce new chemicals and radiation techniques, trying to treat the tumor-filled lungs of smokers on their way to death. Millions are spent for immaculate, intricate, expensive, electronically monitored, tech-nically refined coronary care units for the heart attack victims whose bad eating or smoking habits, stress-filled lifestyles, or lifelong lack of exercise brought them to the crisis. We try to repair and restore the bodies of the accident prone. We buy crutches for the crippled, give tranquilizers to the stressed, provide artificial hearts and hips and kidneys for those whose bodies have broken down.

But we spend very little for the kind of care that will keep people well in the first place. Lifegain proposes to help you change all that.

What Is Lifegain?

Lifegain is a new system for gaining control of your health—and therefore your life—by understanding the influence cultural norms have on your

1

health practices and then changing those norms where needed. Lifegain seeks to help you change your environment to one where your efforts at change can achieve the kind of lasting results that are essential to good health. Lifegain differs from most other programs by its primary emphasis on creating environments where people can achieve sustained success in their efforts at change, rather than giving total attention to the individual change process.

Lifegain's purpose is to change our lifeloss culture to one of lifegain, to change the emphasis from the treatment of disease to the promotion of health, so we can obtain the total wellness we are capable of, but seldom attain.

The Culture Traps

An animal in the woods, whether by instinct or design, bases nearly every action on what is best going to help it survive better and longer. It takes plenty of time out for fun and games but seldom eats or drinks to excess. Nor does it do anything else that is detrimental to its well-being.

When a human baby is born into this world, its instinct, too, is for survival. Even more than babies of other animals, it has complete potential for health and fitness to enjoy its life in the world. But somehow modern-day humans have blown it.

From day one on, the baby's health is chipped away by the negatives of the culture. It is fed sugar and water — setting up the first step in the pattern of bad eating; it is probably separated from its mother unnecessarily, a beginning for stress. It may even have been affected prenatally by drugs, cigarettes, or medicines. Throughout childhood the negative culture works its influences. The child is overfed, enticed to watch television instead of exercising, sees problems handled negatively, learns that speeding is okay, that smoking and drinking are sophisticated, that sleeping is a punishment. In a word, one confronts a negative antihealth culture for its entire lifetime.

Our cultures come in many forms and sizes. Actually, whenever two or more people come together with a shared goal and expected ways of doing things, they form a culture. A culture can be large or small, formally structured or unplanned, can meet regularly or sporadically, can last for a weekend or for generations. A family, a committee, an agency, a hospital, a school, a prison, a corporation, a church, a neighborhood, a city, a police department, a kindergarten, a dormitory, a kingdom — all are examples of cultures. They are all made up of people with some kind of common bond.

A culture — any culture — is comprised of social norms and exerts its power through them. Norms are the behaviors that are expected in a culture, that are accepted and supported by its members. These norms are built up as standards of behavior within the various groups in which we find ourselves — our families, work groups, social circles, communities.

Tomorrow morning try giving your family a salad for breakfast. The comments you get may be of many different kinds — but there surely will be comments, for you will have broken the norm. Or take a jump rope to work and instead of having a coffee break, spend five minutes jumping. Again, the reaction will indicate that you have broken the norm.

A switch of the breakfast menu for one day, a violation of the coffee break norm, probably won't matter too much. But some norms are a matter of life or death.

For example, in many groups it is the norm not to wear seat belts, to drive over the speed limit, to encourage others to eat and drink more than they want, to work long hours without vacations, to have coffee and a roll instead of a nutritional breakfast, to be primarily sports spectators instead of participants.

We live in a culture that shortens our potential lifespan and interferes with our enjoyment of life rather than contributing to it.

These behaviors are more than accidental; they are more than merely individual habits; they are more than just a series of usual happenings. They occur because the culture supports them.

When we really investigate what is going on we find that we are unknowingly being swept along by the norms of our cultures, and these norms are unconsciously influencing our own attitudes toward our bodies, our health practices, our lives. We are swayed so greatly by our surrounding cultures that few of us have made really independent decisions on such critical issues as smoking; eating habits; how we exercise; how we react with our lovers, families, and friends; how we interact at work; how we cope with stress; how we relate to our physicians; or even how we make major life decisions affecting our lives.

As we delve deeper into the cultures that we are a part of and have become so accustomed to — that we have accepted from childhood as "the way things are" — we realize that we are not only destroying our lives but the lives of our children, our loved ones and our friends.

The results? We are slowly killing ourselves because of the way the culture influences our actions.

We are caught in one big culture trap of negative health practices. Until we see that trap, and see it clearly for what it is, we can't begin to get out of it. We can't begin to reach the total health we are capable of.

You have probably seen some of the effects of culture traps yourself. So often, for example, people seem to be just on the verge of feeling good or of finding the meaningful relationships they yearn for, of treating each other better and communicating more, but, except for certain special occasions, some sort of cultural block gets in the way.

On the special occasions, surroundings and circumstances somehow seem to give people permission to behave as they want to. They come together and help when there is a calamity such as a death in the family. Even a snowstorm often brings out friendliness and neighborliness. It seems that people are always on the verge of relating well and when circumstances give them permission, they respond to each other with warmth. But then the old cultural ways move in again.

And in health the same principles prevail. In a group meeting or seminar, or in a burst of personal enthusiasm, people vow to take better care of themselves, to give up smoking, to start exercising, to be more positive mentally. But they soon slide back into the old pattern.

Culture has a strong hold on people.

Psychologists and psychiatrists see the same effects of culture in their practices. They work as therapists in hospitals or private practice doing one-to-one counseling, with the patients improving dramatically. Then they see these good changes in behavior swept away when the person returns to his or her family or social group.

Culture Traps to Watch for in Every Stage of Life

Each stage of life has different peer pressures, different cultural norms, and its own special culture traps. You have to listen and watch as you pass through every stage.

A culture and its traps precede the birth of any individual. We are influenced by our cultures as to whether we have children, how many we have, and how far apart we have them. During pregnancy our culture influences whether we endanger the developing fetus by smoking, drinking, using drugs, not taking vitamin supplements, not eating properly, or not obtaining medical supervision. And our cultures influence what kind of delivery we have, whether the father is present and participates, whether we put the baby in the hospital nursery or stay close to it with rooming-in.

In infancy more culture traps loom: not breast feeding, even though breast feeding may be better for both mother and child; not handling a baby "too much," even though babies who are held and cuddled develop faster physically and mentally; letting the mother do all the child care, instead of also allowing fathers to take an active role in their children's lives.

As the child grows, our cultures continue to determine how we parent. The groups we belong to influence whether we take our children for their physical examinations; whether we get their immunizations; how we treat their trips to the dentist and doctor and their encounters with school; whether we enjoy our parenting or are negative about it; whether we establish healthy behavior patterns for nutrition, exercise, study, recreation; whether we teach them how to get along with others; whether we constantly criticize instead of helping to build self-confidence and a positive self-image. Our cultures determine whether we think every girl should be fragile and every boy should be a he-man and go out for football, or whether we let our children develop their own interests.

As teenagers, the cultures' peer pressures encourage us to prove ourselves in driving, smoking, alcohol, drugs, and sex.

As young adults and in middle age, our cultures give us special stresses of family and job, midlife crises, a sense of failure at not having reached all our life goals, a sense of isolation from others, perhaps sex problems.

In old age we find other culture traps: forced retirement, expectations of mental disability and illness, a sense of uselessness, a denial of sex, society's reluctance to face the reality of death.

But none of these passages needs to be culturally controlled. All of them can be a matter of personal choice and decision. Instead of being culture traps, they can be opportunities for being in charge, making our own decisions. If we are alert to what is happening around us, we can become the creators rather than the victims of our environment. We can choose what we wish, so that we gain life rather than lose it.

The Cost of Our Lifeloss Culture

The cost of our lifeloss culture to us individually and as a nation is staggering. The United States illness bill has surpassed a catastrophic *$200 billion a year!* The United States illness industry is the third largest industry in the nation, with only food and housing using up a larger percentage of the gross national product, and its costs have been estimated to be increasing at the rate of one million dollars an hour. It costs every one of us — man, woman, and child — more than $600 a year whether we use it or not. That's $2,400 for a family of four. And government estimates indicate that it will be twice that in another five years.

And don't think that because your medical and dental expenses are tax deductible, or are paid for by an employer or an insurance company, that they don't really cost you anything. You're still paying for them in the end with higher taxes, higher insurance premiums, and added costs on *all* the products that you buy. One auto company, for example, pays a whopping $825 million in insurance premiums and medical benefits to its employees and estimates this adds $120 to the cost of the car you buy.

What in heaven's name will the cost be to our children if the curve continues?

The human costs of unnecessary suffering and premature deaths are even higher.

We need a commitment to health — a cultural commitment — that supports our individual efforts to stay healthy.

Someday people will look back and marvel about our primitive health practices. We know more about medicine than we ever did before, yet we are not even close to our healthiest.

How many people really feel good?

The lifeloss cultures that we have created for ourselves have become our enemy.

Indeed, to the extent that we even call illness "health," we seem to have let the enemy take over. We have "health" clinics which are really illness clinics, we talk about "health" costs when we really mean illness costs.

Our lifeloss cultures can result in a lot more problems than those of individual illnesses. If a trend were to develop to poorer and poorer health, our inability to alter our health practices could become disastrous to the future of our society and even to the future of the human race.

Change Is Possible

The bee for a millenium has fluttered its wings in the same mating pattern; the social ant also follows its set instinctual patterns. Moths fly to the light, even if it destroys them. We humans, too, have special patterns, but we are different, for we — uniquely — can change our patterns.

Human culture is a two-way business — it creates us, but we can create it. We react to the culture, the culture reacts to us. What is immensely powerful also has tremendous potential for change.

The cultural influence can be positive or negative. We have the flexibility to choose; *we are endowed with the ability to change our behavior patterns if we wish.*

If we use our ability to choose, the massive cultural power could be man's greatest salvation — though at present it seems set more for destruction. We are not making use of our human heritage of being able to decide what our lives could be. We are following along like ants or bees.

The purpose of the Lifegain program and this book is to help you to see why you have made the choices you have in the past, and to help you make the choices you truly want to in the future. It shows you how to find freedom in a presently unfree world.

Lifegain has already shown many people how their health, their lives, and their most vital decisions, were being controlled by forces of which they had little awareness and understanding. Their health — and consequently their happiness — was being controlled more than they had ever suspected by the attitudes of their friends, co-workers, family members, and what our society tells us is the normal way of doing things.

Before starting on the Lifegain steps, some of these people expressed their problems this way:

Mary Browning, weighing 180 pounds: "I don't know why I eat sweets — I know it's bad for me, but I just keep right on doing it. . . . Our family always had big dinners every night and celebrated special occasions with, literally, banquets . . . and when I was good, I was rewarded with candy."

Sally Watson, who was prone to colds and was always tired: "I always thought I didn't exercise because I was lazy. But no one in my circle of friends exercised. When we'd see an occasional person jogging — someone middle-aged like us; it was a big joke. Weirdos, we thought!"

Jim Watson, who was beginning to realize he had a drinking problem: "My parents thought it was cute to let us kids empty out the martini glasses after a party, they had great laughs over our getting drunk."

Joe Graber, a heavy smoker at 21 who had quit smoking four times and started up five times: "All the kids I cared anything about in high school smoked. It was the way to be accepted."

So many of us who think we are free are really not free. Many of our most vital decisions are being controlled by cultural forces. And it often is a shock to learn how much we have not been in control of our decisions and our behavior.

We think we don't exercise because we are lazy, while actually it is because exercise is not expected of us or supported by our friends. If we decided to swim every noon hour at the "Y" instead of having a long, high calorie lunch, we might miss an opportunity to socialize with the people at the office, and we wouldn't feel as much a part of things. If we served light foods at dinnertime, our families might complain.

So what happens is that we usually don't do what's best for us because we don't realize that so many of our vital decisions are being controlled by our culture.

Most of us have made attempts to change — to stop smoking, to take off weight, to reduce stress, to stop being depressed, to get more exercise — but we have tried to do it without understanding the influence of the culture around us, and that is why we have so often failed. For most of us it simply can't be done apart from our cultural environment.

When Mary Browning understood why she was overeating and dealt with the culture she was part of, she was able to lose weight systematically for the first time and to maintain her losses and her new eating practices.

After putting the Lifegain program into practice, Joe Graber was finally able to break through all the previous barriers and stop smoking for good. And as he thought about other problems in his family life, he applied the principles he had learned and found that for the first time he was able to communicate with his family, cooperatively to set some family goals, and actually to have a roaringly good time with his wife and kids.

Sally and Jim Watson were so excited about the results in their own lives that they wanted to spread the word. She got a group started on Lifegain at her office; he encouraged the medical department at his manufacturing plant to set up a program that resulted in saving the company tens of thousands of dollars by decreasing accidents, sick days, and insurance costs and increasing production. And their son Jimmy got another version of it started in his health class at school.

When these people realized how often culture controlled their ideas about things and often set up certain "facts" as accepted and true that were not really true, they were then able to make their own decisions and do things that had never before been possible for them.

This is what we want to do for you in this book. We want to give you a new system to help you take charge of your own body and your own life.

Many of the more traditional efforts have not worked because they haven't sufficiently taken into account the immense power of the culture. Too often our change efforts focus almost exclusively on lectures, workshops, and will-power, neglecting the preparation of the environment. The difference with the Lifegain program is that it pays great attention to creating a supportive environment before beginning the change program and then maintains that environment so that the changes that are made can have deep roots within the culture. In this way Lifegain focuses simultaneously on both the individual and the culture and finds ways for both to work together toward lasting change.

When the gardener plants seeds, he must prepare the ground beforehand and maintain the ground afterward, if he wants the seeds to grow. In the same way, the Lifegain program focuses on the environment for change and maintains the environment necessary for sustained achievement. It is concerned about programs of change, but even more concerned about the environment that exists when the program is introduced, and how a supportive environment can be maintained.

There is a great deal of discussion over whether one program is better than another. For a particular lifestyle change, it has been our Lifegain experience that most programs can succeed if the environment has been prepared beforehand and maintained after the changes have been introduced. And that even good programs often fail if supportive environments are not developed and maintained.

Many of the programs that now exist could be highly successful if the right environment were created for them. With this right environment good health becomes easy. It is no longer a lot of hard work and boring drudgery. It is, in fact, as natural as "being ourselves."

The Lifegain program provides a new way to look at health, a new way to look at all the ways to control fitness, smoking, nutrition, weight, drinking, accidents, stress, and getting along better with people. It will give you a new way to work with your doctor to get to be your healthiest and happiest. It will give you a way to decide for yourself what *you* want.

It gives you a way to become free, to make choices for yourself.

And it gives a way to reach out to others to help them achieve some of these same goals for themselves and for the wider society.

In Lifegain studies, one fact stands out boldly: The cultural norms that surround us are very susceptible to change.

As people in the Lifegain program come to understand cultural influences and how they work, they are able, for the first time in their lives, to decide which of the culture's norms they want to keep, and which they do not want to follow. They find that understanding the cultural base of their individual problem — whether it be smoking, or overweight, or excessive drinking — is the key to making the changes they so badly want.

In this book we are going to give you all of the details of the Lifegain system as it is currently being used. By learning the concepts of the Lifegain program, you will be able to apply the system to your own life, to reach, perhaps for the first time, the total vibrant health you always wanted.

And you will be able to do more to change the cultures around you. Armed with knowledge of cultural norms, you can become a change agent and make things better for your family culture, your work culture, or whatever group you choose to work with.

2 Beyond Illness Medicine

INTRODUCTION

Imagine a society where most people live 10 to 20 years beyond today's usual life expectancy, where the people you meet have a spring in their step and a sense of joy in their lives, where people care about themselves and about one another, where people enjoy life and live it to the fullest.

Such a society is available to us today. It is not something we have to wait for. Our bodies are more than ready for it. And what's more, it wouldn't cost anything. In fact, it could save us billions of dollars.

We satisfy ourselves with what happens to exist when we could have the health we've always dreamed of. And we shall see in this book that the road to a healthy society is actually readily available and need not be too difficult to achieve (Figure 1).

There was a time in human society when we considered it fate if people become sick or died, or we blamed it on angry gods. Gradually the science of curative medicine developed and people began to treat injuries and illness to try to ward off death. For centuries curative medicine was the only medicine, and it is still the traditional kind of medicine practiced today.

Next, physicians and other health specialists became more aware that there were early symptoms or warning signals preceding severe illnesses and that attention to these could sometimes block the progress of the illness and reduce the number of deaths or severe disablements. This was the beginning of preventive medicine.

Even more recently, within the last fifty years and only now with regularity, people began to realize that the early symptoms that were being identified were preceded and often caused by certain negative health practices. Thus, advanced cases of emphysema were preceded by shortness of breath and lung impairment, which in turn may have been preceded by cigarette smoking. In the last ten years there has been an increasing interest in these health practices and in efforts to change them. This has added a new and important dimension to the field of medicine.

All three of these advances have been important ones, and within each area new knowledge and new technology are developing.

However, beyond these is a fourth dimension that thus far has been given little attention despite the fact that it is one more step in the causal relation-

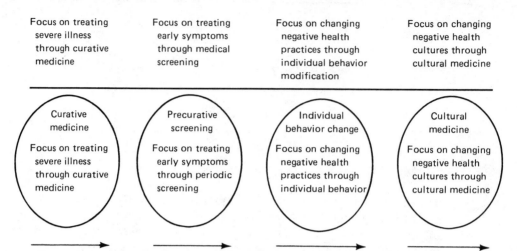

Focus on treating severe illness through curative medicine

Focus on treating early symptoms through medical screening

Focus on changing negative health practices through individual behavior modification

Focus on changing negative health cultures through cultural medicine

Curative medicine

Focus on treating severe illness through curative medicine

Precurative screening

Focus on treating early symptoms through periodic screening

Individual behavior change

Focus on changing negative health practices through individual behavior

Cultural medicine

Focus on changing negative health cultures through cultural medicine

FIGURE 1. Advancing Steps in the History of Prevention of Illness: From Curative Medicine to Cultural Medicine

ship. This fourth dimension—the culture—is the cause of the negative health practices and is the area of one of the major Lifegain focuses.

Traditional medicine has been oriented to treating signs and symptoms after the disease has begun to appear and takes its toll on life and health. Preventive medicine goes before this to try to change things *before* the symptoms appear. The Lifegain approach goes even further than that to *cultural medicine.* Lifegain recognizes the importance of the foregoing—the medical cures, the prevention, and the individual health practices—but it places a new emphasis on treating the culture that causes us to have our poor health practices in the first place. The development of cultural medicine is a logical next step in the advance of medicine.

Lifegain is an application of Normative Systems, a process by which people can change their cultures. Normative Systems has proven its effectiveness as a change mechanism for families, businesses, unions, churches, and community groups, as well as for individuals. In the Lifegain application a person is helped first to determine the factors that may be having a negative impact on his or her health, then to provide an action plan for minimizing those factors and changing them into positive behaviors, and, most importantly, to establish support mechanisms to sustain the changes so they become a natural part of everyday activities. The Lifegain Normative Systems approach gives us a method by which we as individuals can shed the victim's role and change what is "normal."

The result—we can each have the kind of culture that supports our quest for superhealth and can really make preventive medicine work. We can make exercise an essential part of our day, as automatic as brushing our teeth. We can have vibrant energy and joy, can eat right, and can have good relationships with people on an everyday basis.

The culture puts ceilings on our minds to keep us from even trying things that might be possible for us, indeed from even dreaming of them. In Lifegain, people are able to remove the ceilings from their minds.

Dream your wildest dream of how you would like to feel, what you would like your health picture to be. If you get others to join you with their wildest dreams, getting there is not as difficult as you would think.

TOTAL HEALTH

The body is an incredible machine. Most of us just haven't explored our potential. We haven't reached our maximum health, the state of total wellness we could achieve.

Most people think if you are not sick then you must be well. But health is more than the absence of illness.

To be really healthy, totally healthy, is to feel great, to enjoy life, not just to be postponing death and disease.

The next time you are standing on a corner waiting for someone, look around at the people going by. How many of them are glowing with enjoyment, looking fit and healthy, smiling and feeling good? Most people drag their bodies through life. "Imaginary health" one doctor calls it.

The absence of illness is only where health begins. To be healthy is to move out beyond this to where you feel great and look great, to do well whatever you want to do.

That is total wellness. Not just "not sick," but "super well." Not dragging through life half-heartedly; but living it up, operating at your top potential, feeling your best, and having fun.

Traditional medicine only brings a patient to where there is no disease. Lifegain's aim is to take persons beyond the neutral not-sick point to the point of maximum wellness.

When you reach that new state of total wellness, you often find a new satisfaction with your life. You find what so many of us are looking for in life—the feeling of total well-being, exhilaration, a genuine zest for being alive.

You no longer worry too much, eat too much, drink too much, laugh too little, drive too fast. The joy of health is so great you don't need to.

THE SECRETS OF HEALTH AND LONG LIFE IN THE CAUCASUS

Many researchers say the average human lifespan should be about 100 to 110 years. Indeed, all data indicate that when compared to other animals, humans are not living to their full life span. Consider the Hunzas in Soviet

Azerbaijan, an example of a culture with positive health practices. It is common for the Hunzas and several other similar groups of people to continue working, dancing, and being sexually active when 100, some say even 150 years old. (There is some argument about whether the Hunzas truly live to be 150, but even at age 100 their lives are astounding.)

There are now about 19,000 Soviet centenarians. At Kiev's Institute of Gerontology, a branch of the Soviet Academy of Medical Sciences, researchers have been probing the secrets of their long life.

There seem to be a number of factors. These people almost never overeat; they consider it a disgrace and eat with moderation even during high celebrations. They seldom eat candy, sweets, jams, jellies or other sugar, but do eat many garden-fresh, unprocessed fruits and vegetables. They drink wine but not liquor. They laugh easily. They value harmony in personal relationships over wealth, status, and achievement. They start working young and continue into old age. And they have been made to feel socially useful at all ages, both as productive members of a closely knit society and as part of a family. Whether they live in the mountainous Caucasus or in rural areas like Yakutia in Siberia or the Poltaya, Soviet centenarians begin work at 10 or 12 years of age and keep working until retirement at 130 years old or so.

Recently, Soviet physicians gave medical checkups to 40,000 citizens and confirmed that the centenarians among them kept working until an advanced age. As a result, a number of programs are being set up to keep pensioners active, including volunteer jobs. In Kiev, a supervised exercise program was organized three times a week at a local football stadium. Result: senior citizens who exercised, they said, visited the doctor less and had fewer chronic ailments.

It may be only our negative attitudes and habits and the culture that supports them that keep us from reaching the same good health.

What the culture sets up as normal usually determines our everyday health habits. Those health habits usually determine how well and how long we live.

THE BIG EIGHT — THE BIGGEST HEALTH RISKS OF OUR CULTURE

The habits that seem to be the most important in helping us live longer and better are these: being an intelligent eater, staying slim, not smoking, not drinking heavily, getting regular exercise, practicing safety precautions, reducing stress, having good mental health. These are the eight areas on which Lifegain concentrates.

The reason the Big Eight are so important is that they are the factors that have the most influence in reducing risks of people being hit by the biggest killers and cripplers.

The Big Eight largely determine whether you will or will not get heart disease, stroke, cancer, diabetes, or accidents. And these account for more deaths in the United States than all other causes combined. The Big Eight are the culture killers but they can also be the lifesavers. Because they are so important, so central, *the Big Eight are also the most direct route to feeling great and having more enjoyment with total wellness.*

Does changing your Big Eight habits really help? You can bet your life it does!

The average person can easily add eight years to life, say insurance companies, by simply keeping blood pressure and cholesterol levels down, drinking moderately or not at all, not smoking, exercising, and maintaining normal weight.

In fact, according to the U.S. Public Health Service, in the United States today at least 53 percent of deaths are caused by lifestyle, not body defects.

And if you work on all of the Big Eight, not just one, it's even better because they don't just add on to each other in their effect, they *multiply!* For example, if you are between the ages of 30 and 59 and have high blood pressure, your risk of dying of a major disease in the next ten years is more than twice that of a person who doesn't have high blood pressure. If you also smoke *and* have high cholesterol, your risk of death is *five* times higher. If you are overweight, getting your weight down to normal will also reduce your risk of heart attack, stroke, and diabetes.

The Big Eight definitely control your chances of being attacked by the big killers and cripplers. Working with just the Big Eight and nothing else can change your entire health picture.

A striking demonstration of the effect health habits can have on health was found in a study conducted by Dr. Nedra B. Belloc and Dr. Lester Breslow of the California State Department of Public Health at UCLA's Department of Preventive and Social Medicine. They studied 7,000 people in several small California communities to determine what influences good health and what does not. The Belloc-Breslow study showed that those people's health was definitely affected by their sleep habits, eating habits, amount of exercise, whether they smoked cigarettes, or drank excessively. Each of the factors was important, they found, and if a person followed good habits in all of the categories the effect toward good health multiplied. And astoundingly, they reported that the average physical health status of those over age 75 who followed all of the good practices was the same as those age 35 to 44 who followed fewer than three of the good health practices. They concluded that a lifetime of good health practices appears to produce good health and extends the period of good health status by some 30 years!

A follow-up study five years later on the same people showed that the health habits also affected how long they lived. Those following three or less of the good health practices had a death rate four times higher than those who practiced seven good habits. A 45-year-old man who followed seven of the good health habits could be expected to live a good 33 years more compared to only 21 years for the 45-year-old man who practiced only three or less of the habits.

So we really can live longer and better. We can control the risks around us. We can have a culture as healthy as that of the Hunzas.

In the following chapters we will outline a system with specific techniques for changing your environment so that you can increase your lifespan and improve the quality of your life.

But first let's look at how Lifegain began.

HOW IT ALL BEGAN

Our first clear look at the immense power of the culture over people's lives took place more than 20 years ago as we were studying the development of delinquent behavior patterns in northern ghettos. As a young social scientist, the senior author of this book took up residence in a ghetto area in New York City where an amazing phenomenon was occurring. Young men were arriving from the rural South never having been engaged in delinquency in their lives. Six months later they were appearing in the children's courts of the city with all the skills of full-fledged delinquents. Here indeed was a remarkable training program! It occurred to us that we might be able to harness this same cultural power in the cause of their freedom.

The project that resulted proved that people could break out of their culture traps and change their lives, that they could substitute positive ways for negative ways, and learn to redesign their worlds. It was the beginning of the development of the Normative Systems change process.

It Takes a System to Beat a System

That's what people were learning. The power of any negative culture was strong and the only way to break from its trap was with a stronger positive culture and an awareness of what was occurring. You could put culture to work *for* you as well as against you. Other applications followed in rapid succession.

One was an exciting project with migrant workers in Florida, a group of seemingly helpless, victimized people. But the company they worked for and the people themselves succeeded in setting up an entire new dignified manner of living. Juan was one of the people. All his life Juan had picked oranges in the groves in central Florida, maintaining only a marginal existence. Today he is still an orange picker, but he works year round, owns his own home, makes a comfortable living, has hospitals, clinics, daycare centers, libraries, and schools available for himself and his children.

Both of these projects rose out of cultures that were mired (hopelessly, the people thought at the time) in whole systems of expected behaviors that had kept people from achieving what they wanted. They only had to discover their own power together to make change.

Soon the system was being used in many situations, in groups ranging from small family units to large corporations, schools, and communities. Wherever it was used it was shown to be a system for freeing people from the restrictions that their cultures had placed upon them. The primary aim, no matter what the application, was to help people find a way to help themselves, to determine the course of their lives.

The system was applied to such problems as environmental care, organizational teamwork, litter, equal employment opportunity, and even conflict resolution between police and ghetto residents.

The Lifegain program was a natural outgrowth of more than 600 applications to a variety of different problems.

Human Resources Institute and the Lifegain Program

As enthusiasm grew, an institute was set up — The Human Resources Institute. At The Human Resources Institute, behavioral scientists, psychologists, and related professionals attempted to apply all these new concepts on a more formal basis, working with businesses, unions, schools, and government and voluntary agencies as well as with small groups and individuals.

As with other Human Resource Institute projects, the Lifegain program began with a careful analysis of the kinds of cultures that were influencing people's lives and then proceeded to small pilot programs in a variety of settings: schools, businesses, families, and communities. As these pilot programs developed, people for the first time began to break out of their health culture traps, and many of the participants found they could make their own decisions about their health.

People began to look at their lives from a cultural perspective. They began to understand how their health decisions had really been decided by their cultures. If they grew up in a culture where poor health habits were emphasized, they were apt to flow right into that same negative pattern. And they began to realize that the cultural norms that they had adopted were not really the norms they would usually have chosen for themselves if given the chance. They began to see that they ate, drank, worried, and smoked too much; drove too fast; and behaved in other ways that threatened health. And they realized they wanted a change.

Gradually, aware of what the culture was doing, they were able to free themselves. People who had not been able to lose weight found that now they could. People who had not been able to stop smoking found it possible to stop and stay stopped. People who had been too embarrassed to get out and exercise or to practice accident prevention found now they could make the decision they really wanted to make, and they did it.

They found they enjoyed food more, enjoyed people more, enjoyed their jobs more, enjoyed sex more, and enjoyed themselves and their families more. And many people also reported a reduction in doctor and medical bills and said they missed less time at work because of illness, were accomplishing more, and felt more capable of living their lives more fully.

Before being interested in Lifegain, people found they had been playing the health game with all the cards stacked against them. Now, with understanding, they were in control of their own lives and health and could play the game the way they wanted to.

3 Checking Your Personal and Cultural Health Status

What are your own personal health habits? What do you eat? How much do you exercise, smoke, or drink? How much do you weigh? How safety-conscious are you? How well do you control stress, get along with yourself and others? These are the chief hazards to your personal health and the chief avenues by which you can reach total wellness in the shortest time.

By knowing where you stand in each of these areas, you can change your health practices where necessary to prevent simple bad habits from becoming major problems that can cripple your lifestyle or bring you closer to death.

In this book we cannot be your doctor and give you a physical examination. Nor can we be a computer to feed in hundreds of answers about your lifestyle. But we can help you to start assessing your own health and the quality of your life. The self-analytical questions in this chapter will help you identify those elements in your life that contribute to your general health profile and those that are hazardous and need correcting. Since your cultural situation is an important part of you and cannot be ignored in an assessment of where you are in regard to your health, a questionnaire concerning cultural influences (Health Practices Norm Indicator) is also included.

The answers you give in these analyses then will help you plan your own customized Lifegain program to obtain the maximum benefits and highest payoffs in total health for your own life.

HOW TO CALCULATE YOUR LIFE EXPECTANCY

While there is no sure way to calculate your life expectancy even with computer systems, there are certain guidelines, such as this test, that can give you rough estimates. If you are age 20 to 65 and reasonably healthy, this test provides a life insurance company's statistical view of your life expectancy.

Start with the number 72.

Personal Data:
   If you are male, subtract three.
   If female, add four.

If you live in an urban area with a population over two million, subtract two.

If you live in a town under 10,000 or on a farm, add two.

If a grandparent lived to 85, add two.

If all four grandparents lived to 80, add six.

If either parent died of a stroke or heart attack before the age of 50, subtract four.

If any parent, brother, or sister under 50 has (or had) cancer or a heart condition, or has had diabetes since childhood, subtract three.

Do you earn over $50,000 a year? Subtract two.

If you finished college, add one. If you have a graduate or professional degree, add two more.

If you are 65 or over and still working, add three.

If you live with a spouse or friend, add five. If not, subtract one for every 10 years alone since age 25.

Healthstyle facts:

If you work behind a desk, subtract three.

If your work requires regular, heavy physical labor, add three.

If you exercise strenuously (tennis, running, swimming, etc.) five times a week for at least a half-hour, add four. Two or three times a week, add two.

Do you sleep more than 10 hours each night? Subtract four.

Are you intense, aggressive, easily angered? Subtract three.

Are you easygoing and relaxed? Add three.

Are you happy? Add one. Unhappy? Subtract two.

Have you had a speeding ticket in the last year? Subtract one.

Do you smoke more than two packs a day? Subtract eight. One to two packs? Subtract six. One-half to one? Subtract three.

Do you drink the equivalent of a quart bottle of liquor a day? Subtract one.

Are you overweight by 50 pounds or more? Subtract eight. By 30 to 50 pounds? Subtract four. By 10 to 30 pounds? Subtract two.

If you are a man over 40 and have annual checkups, add two.

If you are a woman and see a gynecologist once a year, add two.

Age adjustment:

If you are between 30 and 40, add two.

If you are between 40 and 50, add three.

If you are between 50 and 70, add four.

If you are over 70, add five.

Add up your score to get your life expectancy at this time. Now compare it to the national average for various ages:

Age Now	Male	Female
0–10	69.8	77.2
11–19	70.3	77.5
20–29	71.2	77.8
30–39	71.3	77.9
40–49	73.5	79.4
50–59	76.1	79.0
60–69	80.2	83.6
70–79	85.9	87.7
80–90	90.0	91.1

If you would like your life expectancy to come out at a later age, look back over the questions relating to health practices and find those in which you subtracted years. Change those to positive health practices and you can add many years to your life expectancy.

HOW TO DETERMINE YOUR OWN MOST MAJOR RISKS

What are the major killers for your age level? What are the most important things statistically you have to look out for? And how well are you protecting yourself against them?

Look over this list of national averages of leading causes of death to find your biggest potential enemies (Tables 1 and 2).

In figuring your own path to the best health, you also need to consider your past medical history and your family's medical history. If your parents died young of heart disease, you would choose programs especially good for reducing risks of heart disease: diet, smoking, and stress chapters. If you have high blood pressure, you might want to work especially on the Lifegain programs on nutrition, weight loss, exercise, and stress. Or if you have an ulcer, learning stress control might give you the biggest payoff.*

ARE YOU REACHING YOUR FULL HUMAN POTENTIAL?

Good health is not just the absence of illness or the number of years lived. It is the full realization of our potential as human beings in our family, our

*If you would like a more complete, computerized assessment of your health risks, you may want to contact Dr. Lewis Robbins, Methodist Hospital, 1604 N. Capitol Avenue, Indianapolis, Indiana 46202; or Dr. William Hettler, University of Wisconsin Health Services, Stevens Point, Wisconsin. Dr. Robbins is one of the foremost leaders in this field and his book, *How To Practice Prospective Medicine*, is the "Bible" in the health hazard appraisal area. Dr. Hettler is also one of the top leaders in this field and his Life-style Assessment Inventory is one of the best that is presently available.

TABLE 1. Leading Causes of Death: Male

AGE	WHITE		BLACK	
	CAUSE	*PERCENT*	*CAUSE*	*PERCENT*
15–19	1. Auto accidents	43.5	1. Homicide	22.4
	2. Suicide	6.1	2. Auto accidents	22.1
	3. Drowning	4.7	3. Drowning	9.4
	4. Homicide	3.5	4. Firearms accidents	3.1
	5. Firearms accidents	2.8	5. Pneumonia	2.4
20–24	1. Auto accidents	36.8	1. Homicide	25.6
	2. Suicide	7.8	2. Auto accidents	19.5
	3. Homicide	4.0	3. Drowning	4.3
	4. Drowning	2.5	4. Suicide	3.1
	5. Aircraft accidents	2.5	5. Pneumonia	2.6
25–29	1. Auto accidents	23.7	1. Homicide	23.2
	2. Suicide	9.0	2. Auto accidents	12.7
	3. Heart attack	6.2	3. Heart attack	4.2
	4. Homicide	3.5	4. Pneumonia	3.6
	5. Rheumatic heart	2.5	5. Suicide	3.4
30–34	1. Heart attack	15.5	1. Homicide	16.3
	2. Auto accidents	14.2	2. Heart attack	8.9
	3. Suicide	8.4	3. Auto accidents	8.2
	4. Cirrhosis	3.2	4. Pneumonia	4.6
	5. Rheumatic heart	3.0	5. Stroke	4.6
35–39	1. Heart attack	26.2	1. Heart attack	12.2
	2. Auto accidents	8.5	2. Homicide	10.1
	3. Suicide	6.8	3. Stroke	6.2
	4. Cirrhosis	4.0	4. Auto accidents	5.8
	5. Stroke	3.6	5. High blood pressure	5.2
40–44	1. Heart attack	33.8	1. Heart attack	15.9
	2. Auto accidents	5.1	2. Stroke	8.8
	3. Suicide	4.7	3. High blood pressure	6.6
	4. Cirrhosis	4.0	4. Homicide	6.2
	5. Stroke	4.0	5. Pneumonia	5.0
45–49	1. Heart attack	37.9	1. Heart attack	19.2
	2. Cancer (lungs)	5.2	2. Stroke	10.6
	3. Stroke	4.6	3. High blood pressure	7.0
	4. Cirrhosis	4.0	4. Pneumonia	4.4
	5. Suicide	3.4	5. Cancer (lungs)	4.0
50–54	1. Heart attack	40.2	1. Heart attack	21.1
	2. Cancer (lungs)	6.0	2. Stroke	12.1
	3. Stroke	5.0	3. High blood pressure	7.6
	4. Cirrhosis	3.4	4. Cancer (lungs)	4.6
	5. Suicide	2.4	5. Pneumonia	4.0
55–59	1. Heart attack	41.0	1. Heart attack	23.2
	2. Stroke	6.2	2. Stroke	13.6
	3. Cancer (lungs)	6.0	3. High blood pressure	8.0
	4. Cancer (colon)	2.6	4. Cancer (lungs)	4.4
	5. Cirrhosis	2.4	5. Pneumonia	4.0

TABLE 1 (Continued)

AGE	WHITE			BLACK		
	CAUSE		PERCENT	CAUSE		PERCENT
60-64	1. Heart attack		40.4	1. Heart attack		24.0
	2. Stroke		8.2	2. Stroke		14.5
	3. Cancer (lungs)		5.4	3. High blood pressure		8.5
	4. Cancer (colon)		3.0	4. Pneumonia		4.0
	5. High blood pressure		2.6	5. Cancer (stomach)		4.0
65-69	1. Heart attack		39.4	1. Heart attack		24.6
	2. Stroke		10.7	2. Stroke		15.6
	3. Cancer (lungs)		4.4	3. High blood pressure		8.4
	4. High blood pressure		3.0	4. Pneumonia		4.0
	5. Cancer (colon)		3.0	5. Cancer (prostate)		3.6
70-74	1. Heart attack		38.4	1. Heart attack		25.0
	2. Stroke		13.2	2. Stroke		16.5
	3. High blood pressure		3.6	3. High blood pressure		8.0
	4. Arterial disease		3.6	4. Pneumonia		4.5
	5. Pneumonia		3.0	5. Cancer (prostate)		4.0

Adopted from: Health Hazard Appraisal Program, Methodist Hospital, Indianapolis.

TABLE 2. Leading Causes of Death: Female

AGE	WHITE			BLACK		
	CAUSE		PERCENT	CAUSE		PERCENT
15-19	1. Auto accidents		28.2	1. Homicide		10.9
	2. Suicide		4.2	2. Auto accidents		9.1
	3. Pneumonia		4.0	3. Rheumatic heart		4.0
	4. Congenital circu-			4. Pneumonia		3.8
	latory defects		3.5	5. Stroke		3.6
	5. Leukemia		2.9			
20-24	1. Auto accidents		18.0	1. Homicide		11.4
	2. Suicide		6.1	2. Auto accidents		6.8
	3. Rheumatic heart		4.1	3. Stroke		5.2
	4. Stroke		3.5	4. Pneumonia		4.3
	5. Cancer (lymphatic)		3.0	5. Tuberculosis		4.0
25-29	1. Auto accidents		10.7	1. Homicide		9.2
	2. Suicide		7.0	2. Stroke		6.6
	3. Rheumatic heart		5.0	3. Pneumonia		5.0
	4. Stroke		4.1	4. Heart attack		4.2
	5. Cancer (breast)		3.7	5. Tuberculosis		4.0
30-34	1. Cancer (breast)		7.5	1. Stroke		7.6
	2. Auto accidents		7.2	2. Homicide		6.2
	3. Suicide		5.8	3. Heart attack		6.2
	4. Rheumatic heart		5.0	4. High blood pressure		5.8
	5. Stroke		4.6	5. Cancer (cervix)		4.5

TABLE 2   (Continued)

AGE	WHITE		BLACK	
	CAUSE	*PERCENT*	*CAUSE*	*PERCENT*
35–39	1. Cancer (breast)	10.3	1. Stroke	9.8
	2. Heart attack	6.8	2. Heart attack	8.8
	3. Stroke	5.6	3. High blood pressure	8.2
	4. Rheumatic heart	5.0	4. Cancer (cervix)	4.8
	5. Cancer (cervix)	4.8	5. Cancer (breast)	4.6
40–44	1. Cancer (breast)	11.6	1. Heart attack	12.3
	2. Heart attack	9.8	2. Stroke	12.2
	3. Stroke	6.6	3. High blood pressure	9.6
	4. Cancer (cervix)	4.5	4. Cancer (breast)	5.0
	5. Rheumatic heart	4.4	5. Cancer (cervix)	4.5
45–49	1. Heart attack	13.4	1. Heart attack	15.2
	2. Cancer (breast)	11.4	2. Stroke	14.2
	3. Stroke	7.6	3. High blood pressure	10.6
	4. Cancer (colon)	4.6	4. Cancer (breast)	4.4
	5. Rheumatic heart	4.0	5. Cancer (cervix)	3.8
50–54	1. Heart attack	19.2	1. Heart attack	17.1
	2. Cancer (breast)	9.2	2. Stroke	16.2
	3. Stroke	8.0	3. High blood pressure	11.6
	4. Cancer (colon)	5.0	4. Cancer (breast)	3.4
	5. High blood pressure	3.6	5. Cancer (cervix)	2.7
55–59	1. Heart attack	25.7	1. Heart attack	20.2
	2. Stroke	9.2	2. Stroke	18.2
	3. Cancer (breast)	6.8	3. High blood pressure	12.0
	4. Cancer (colon)	5.0	4. Cancer (breast)	2.4
	5. High blood pressure	4.0	5. Cancer (colon)	2.4
60–64	1. Heart attack	30.4	1. Heart attack	21.5
	2. Stroke	11.2	2. Stroke	19.5
	3. Cancer (breast)	4.8	3. High blood pressure	12.0
	4. High blood pressure	4.6	4. Pneumonia	2.5
	5. Cancer (colon)	4.4	5. Cancer (uterus)	2.1
65–69	1. Heart attack	32.2	1. Heart attack	23.1
	2. Stroke	13.8	2. Stroke	20.0
	3. High blood pressure	5.6	3. High blood pressure	11.4
	4. Cancer (colon)	4.0	4. Pneumonia	3.0
	5. Cancer (breast)	3.4	5. Arterial disease	2.6
70–74	1. Heart attack	34.0	1. Heart attack	24.0
	2. Stroke	16.8	2. Stroke	20.5
	3. High blood pressure	6.0	3. High blood pressure	10.1
	4. Cancer (colon)	3.4	4. Arterial disease	3.0
	5. Pneumonia	2.6	5. Pneumonia	3.0

Adopted from: Health Hazard Appraisal Program, Methodist Hospital, Indianapolis.

work, our community, and the world. It involves not just feeling well and looking well but also the enjoyment of life, the ability to develop caring relationships, and it involves our capacity for contributing to the world in which we live and for making it the kind of place we and our children want and need.

Avoiding illness is only half the battle, and good health is poorly used if it does not enable us to do the things we want to do and to make a contribution to our society. This living to our full potential as human beings is a central concept of the Lifegain program.

Quality of Life Test

As you look at your present personal health practice, rate yourself from 1 to 5 in the following areas:

	Living up to my full potential	Doing well	Needs some improvement	Needs major improvement	Not acceptable
How am I doing:					
1. In my work	5	4	3	2	1
2. In enjoying myself as opposed to being bored or angry	5	4	3	2	1
3. In my relationships with others	5	4	3	2	1
4. In expressing my emotions when I want to	5	4	3	2	1
5. In my use and enjoyment of my leisure time	5	4	3	2	1
6. In my sexual relationships	5	4	3	2	1
7. In what I accomplish during the day	5	4	3	2	1
8. In having enough fun	5	4	3	2	1
9. In making use of the talents that I have	5	4	3	2	1
10. In achieving my own health potential, feeling physically tops and full of vitality	5	4	3	2	1
11. In developing my skills and abilities	5	4	3	2	1
12. In contributing to my society	5	4	3	2	1

	Living up to my full potential	Doing well	Needs some improvement	Needs major improve- ment	Not acceptable

How am I doing:

13. In being helpful to other people	5	4	3	2	1
14. In having a sense of free- dom and adventure in life	5	4	3	2	1
15. In having a sense of joy and pleasure on most days	5	4	3	2	1
16. In having an exuberant sense of fitness that my body can meet demands put upon it	5	4	3	2	1
17. In feeling rested and full of energy	5	4	3	2	1
18. In being able to relax most of the day	5	4	3	2	1
19. In enjoying a good night's sleep	5	4	3	2	1
20. In usually going to bed feeling happy and satisfied about the day	5	4	3	2	1

How high was your score compared with a potential score of 100? This will give you an estimate of the usual quality of your life.

Could it be improved?

In what areas?

And just as culture can negatively influence our health practices, it can negatively influence our human potential, putting a kind of ceiling on our minds that keeps us from becoming all that we are capable of being.

Assessing Your Cultural Situation

The following Survey of Cultural Influences will help you to review the impact of your culture upon your health practices and to what extent your culture is supportive of your efforts. These norms are an important part of you, for it is not only *you* but *you-in-your-culture* that determines your health.

The following are the attitudes and norms frequently found in our families, social groups, organizations, and communities. This questionnaire is designed to identify some of the key norms that may be influencing your own health-related behavior. Read through the list, and put a check mark before each norm that exists in one or more of the groups that you belong to.

Remember, you are not being asked how you think it should be but rather how you see it "as it really is" in the groups you are in contact with.

A CULTURAL NORM INDICATOR: IT IS A NORM IN ONE OR MORE GROUPS THAT I BELONG TO:

Exercise

1. for people not to exercise as much as would be healthy for them.
2. for people to use their cars to go short distances even when there is no need to do so.
3. for people to look upon exercise as a grind rather than as a source of pleasure.
4. for people to be surprised when someone uses the stairs instead of the elevator or escalator.
5. for people to spend more time watching sports than they do participating in them.
6. for people not to make exercise a regular part of their daily lives.

Smoking Norms

7. for people to smoke cigarettes, cigars, and pipes to the extent that it is a hazard to their health.
8. for people to feel that the illness and death statistics regarding smoking will somehow not apply to them.
9. for smoking to be presented as a desirable behavior in newspaper and magazine ads.
10. for young people to smoke because it is the thing to do.
11. for people to smoke without asking others present if it is all right to do so.
12. for people to smoke in public buildings and restaurants, even in closed rooms or cars when other people are present.
13. for people not to mention it if someone else's smoking bothers them.

Stress Norms

14. for people to take on more responsibility than they can handle.
15. for people to avoid asking for help if their work load becomes too heavy.
16. for people not to understand the harmful effects that continued stress can have upon their health.
17. for people to look upon stress as something that they can't do anything about.
18. for people to accept high tension levels in their lives, thinking that is the way life is.

Weight Control Norms

19. for people to eat more food than they want or need.
20. for people to look at being slightly overweight as "natural," particularly among older people.
21. for people not to balance their food intake with their physical exercise as they grow older.
22. for people to see children who are slightly overweight as healthier and better cared for than children who aren't.
23. for people to see desserts such as cake, pie, pudding, and ice cream as an expected part of a lunch or dinner menu.
24. for sweets to be thought of as special treats and therefore more "rewarding" than more nutritious foods.
25. for parents to encourage children to clean up all the food on their plates even if it is more than they want or need.
26. for people to associate overindulging in food with relaxation, pleasure, and good social relationships.
27. for hosts and hostesses to encourage guests to eat more food than would be desirable for them.

Nutrition Norms

28. for people to pay very little attention to the nutritional value of the foods that they eat.
29. for people to have coffee and a roll instead of a nutritional breakfast in the morning.
30. for people to drink a great many coffee and cola drinks and other caffeine-based beverages.
31. for people to think of people who pay attention to nutrition as "health nuts."
32. for people not to get a balance of meat, fruits, vegetables, milk, and carbohydrates in their daily diet.
33. for people not to have sufficient information about nutrition and its impact on health.

Alcohol and Alcohol Abuse Norms

34. for the host or hostess at a party to check repeatedly to make sure everyone's glass is full and drinks are being continually replenished.
35. to persuade guests to stay for one more round or have one more for the road.
36. to mention with pride one's own ability or a friend's ability to consume large amounts of alcohol.
37. to have a drink when one doesn't really want to, just because the others are.
38. for the use of alcohol to be presented as the "in thing" to do in magazines and TV advertisements.
39. for young people to be encouraged to drink by their peers.

40. for people to offer their guests a drink at most social gatherings in the home.
41. for waiters and waitresses and others in restaurants to "expect" that people will be having a drink before or during dinner.
42. for people who don't drink at a social gathering to be looked upon as not having as much fun as those who do.

Safety Norms

43. for people to look upon safety rules and regulations as something for others to follow — not themselves.
44. for people to think it's OK to drive over the posted speed limit so long as they are not caught.
45. for people not to wear seat belts when they feel it is inconvenient to do so.
46. for people to drive when drowsy or under the influence of alcohol or medications.
47. for people to leave pills and other dangerous or poisonous materials around the house in places that might be easily accessible to children.
48. for people to ignore safety hazards or violations rather than seeing that they are corrected.

Mental Health Norms

49. for people to keep feelings bottled up inside rather than to express them openly.
50. for people to see mental health problems as something to be ashamed of and hidden.
51. for people to hold off seeking help with emotional problems until they become very severe.
52. for people to hold back on expressing positive feelings in their relationships with others.
53. for people to be less effective in their human relations skills than they might be.
54. for people not to handle conflict situations with other people constructively.
55. for people to let problems become chronic rather than dealing with them promptly and constructively.
56. for people not to achieve an adequate balance between work, rest, and play in their lives.
57. for people to bury their creative urges and talents.
58. for people not to see themselves as being as capable as they really are.
59. for people not to have as much enjoyment in their lives as they are capable of having.
60. for people to work so hard that they tend to lose contact with other important parts of their lives, e.g., their children, their friends, other interests, etc.

How many of the above norms did you check as being present in one or more of the groups that you belong to? If you are like most of us, it was probably a large number, and it is these norms that you will need to take into account in planning your own change program.

Assessing Your Present Health Practices

As we have seen, there are a number of health practices that can affect the length and quality of our lives. Some of the most important of these are shown in the Health Practices Assessment Inventory that follows.

HEALTH PRACTICES ASSESSMENT INVENTORY

1. *Smoking* Do you smoke? Yes —— No ——
Number per day: Cigarettes —— Cigars —— Pipes ——

2. *Exercise* How many days a week do you vigorously exercise for at least 20 minutes? 0 —— 1 —— 2 —— 3 —— 4 —— 5 —— 6 —— 7 ——
How physically active are you? Very active —— Active —— Moderate —— Inactive ——

3. *Driving Safety* What percentage of the time do you wear seat belts? 100% —— 75% —— 50% —— 25% —— 0% ——
What percentage of the time do you drive more than five miles over the speed limit? 100% —— 75% —— 50% —— 25% —— 0% ——

4. *Alcohol* How many alcoholic drinks (including wine or beer) do you drink in an average day? ——

5. *Weight and Height* What is your weight? —— Height? ——
Number of pounds overweight/underweight. 0 —— 5 —— 10 —— 15 —— 20 —— 25 —— 30 —— 35 ——

6. *Nutrition* How many days per week do you eat a well-balanced breakfast? 0 —— 1 —— 2 —— 3 —— 4 —— 5 —— 6 —— 7 ——
How frequently do you maintain a nutritious, well-balanced eating pattern? All of the time —— Most of the time —— Some of the time —— Seldom —— Not at all ——
Circle those items that you consistently limit in your daily diet: Salt Sugar Fats Caffeine

7. *Stress* How would you rate the level of stress in your life at the present time? Very high —— High —— Moderate —— Low —— Very low ——
How would you rate the effectiveness with which you deal with stress on a regular basis? Excellent —— Very well —— Well —— Only fair —— Poorly ——

8. *Mental Health*

To what extent are you able to maintain a positive, healthy outlook on life? Always —— Almost always —— Sometimes —— Seldom ——

To what extent are you able to make a significant contribution to the life of others? Always —— Almost always ——

You now have an idea about which areas to concentrate on to give yourself the greatest chance to live longer, to be healthier, to look and feel better, and live a fuller life.

You are now beginning to see your strengths and weaknesses, what life patterns you should continue and which ones you have the opportunity to improve upon.

Reaching the good health you want isn't really that difficult or complicated. There are many refinements that you can make, but the basic program to good health is really only a few do's and don'ts.

Do eat nutritious food; do exercise adequately; do practice safety precautions at home, at work, and on the road; do learn to relax and cope with stress; do build positive relationships with others. Don't smoke; don't misuse alcohol; don't become overweight.

Step by step in a few weeks you can begin to see changes over the habits of many years. And soon you can take charge of your own life and help determine how long and how well you wish to live.

4 — Taking Charge of Your Life and Health

A recent survey of health attitudes in a large city showed that good health was held to be *the* most important thing in life by the large majority of people questioned.

We value good health, yet we practice self-destructive behaviors that are injurious to our health. It's pretty obvious when you shorten your life by suicide; but alcoholism, heavy smoking, severe stress, eating too much, exercising too little can be just as lethal as suicide.

An anthropologist in the future looking back on our culture would shake his head in disbelief at all the things we are doing in our culture to make ourselves sick. As a result of the culture, many people find themselves firmly acting out a death wish. What we need to do is create cultures that cultivate a life wish. If our life is really worth something to us, and hopefully it is, it should be worth saving.

You don't have to keep killing yourself just because the rest of the culture does. Instead you can reach toward the total wellness you have always wanted.

SHEDDING THE VICTIM'S ROLE

Elephants in India are chained to pegs when they are very young and weak. Day by day they grow bigger and stronger, until they could easily snap the pegs that hold them and walk off. But they never realize this and docilely walk their narrow circles, held back from freedom only by their illusions.

We are often like the self-trapped elephants, held back by our perceptions. We feel powerless while actually we have at our disposal tremendous energy for change. The realization that our chains can be broken is the first step toward snapping them.

The biggest hurdle is to recognize the greatest culture trap of all, the feeling that you can't change because "It's just human nature;" "That's the way it is;" "You can't fight it;" "Nobody has ever done it."

Actually, very few things in human nature are as limited as we would believe. An illustration — the four-minute mile. For years runners had tried to break the record, but nobody had been able to run the mile in less than four minutes. It seemed to be the limitation of the human body until Roger Bannister came along. On May 6, 1954, in Oxford, England, he ran the mile in 3 minutes, 59.4 seconds and broke through an invisible barrier. Soon after, several more runners broke the four-minute record. Now sub-four-minute miles have become almost commonplace. What had seemed to be a physiological barrier turned out to be a psychological one. When no one believed it could be done, it wasn't done.

It's Easier To Do Than You Think

The failures that people experience in bringing about lasting change in their lives are less a result of people's resistance to change than they are the result of the lack of effectiveness of the change processes that they employ.

Working with the change process described in this book, lifelong cigarette smokers who had earlier given up hope of kicking the habit have given up cigarettes for good. Ten-time losers in the United States weight reduction marathon have not only lost the unwanted pounds but have permanently changed their eating habits and food preferences. Similarly, people have made lasting changes in their exercise habits, drinking patterns, and stress management practices. An what is more, they have had fun and enjoyment doing it.

To be sure, it has taken commitment and effort, and there have been some difficult times, but as one Lifegain group member put it, "While sometimes it has not been quite so easy as I had wished, it has never been nearly so difficult as I had thought it would be."

One of the first things that needs to be done is to raise our "culture consciousness." Being alert to the influences of the culture, you begin to recognize the signs of it in your everyday life. You learn to hear the click of the culture traps. "Come on Bill, don't be a square." *Click*. "Come on, Mary, everybody's doing it." *Click*. Soon you can begin to recognize how cultural norms influence your own health related behaviors in such areas as exercise, smoking, drinking, weight, nutrition, accidents, stress, mental health, even in how you get along with your doctor. And with the flash of recognition, you pause to think it through, then do what *you* want to do. Soon it becomes easier to make your own decisions about your life and your lifestyle.

In the Lifegain studies, one fact stands out boldly: Our own lifestyle practices and the cultural norms that influence them *are* susceptible to change. In fact, they can be changed amazingly quickly *if* we approach the change process in a creative and systematic way.

True Freedom

So many people who think they are free are really not free. They are still caught in a culture trap. The adolescent who thinks he is free of his parents and smokes to prove it, has just picked up another brand of conformity, the conformity to a culture that says it's smart to smoke.

True freedom is more than merely following the culture's dictates. It is a matter of making our own choices for ourselves. This does not mean that we can ever be completely free of our cultures, nor would we want to be. But we can be free to choose and design the cultures we actually want. We can be free of the cultures' blind power over us, free of having our decisions unknowingly controlled by powers of culture that we are largely unaware of. Instead, we can purposefully design our futures to be healthier, more rewarding, more satisfying, and more fun.

No other species can take charge of its life with conscious decision making as humans can. We are uniquely in charge of our own destinies, including our health.

In the final analysis, we can do with our bodies what we choose to do. When we choose, we can choose knowingly, aware of the impact of culture upon us, and shaping its influence to our own needs and purposes.

THE SEVEN STEPS OF LIFEGAIN

In working with people on the implementation of change programs over a period of years, we have identified seven interrelated steps that have proven helpful in bringing about sustained lifestyle improvements. These steps, when creatively and flexibly applied to one's own change priorities, can provide the basis for successful, individual change. While they are listed in a sequential order, it is not necessary that you follow that order if some other seems more comfortable for you. It probably will be useful, however, if all of the steps are included, since the neglect of any one of them could get in the way of the long-range achievements that you are looking to accomplish.

Step One. Understand Your Culture

As we have seen, our cultures tend to have a very strong negative impact upon our health practices. If we wish to change and to maintain health changes for any length of time, we need to become aware of this impact and to arrange our lives in such a way that the negative influences are minimal and positive influences are substituted for them.

In working out your own change process, you will find that it is not usually necessary for you drastically to change the wider cultures that surround you, but it is important that you take them into account and plan for avoiding the pitfalls that they may present. To paraphrase the statement, "Those who do not understand history may live to repeat it," we might say that "Those who do not understand their cultures may live to be negatively influenced by them."

Step One helps you to identify the norms of the negative cultures that may be affecting you, so you can recognize the culture traps in the expectations of your family, friends, co-workers, and other groups influencing you. The light bulb clicks on in your brain as you recognize the culture traps for what they are.

By recognizing these influences, you can systematically deal with them so you no longer find yourself swimming upstream in the face of the culture.

In Step One you study your own culture and determine which factors are having a negative pull on your life and which are positive. The positive norms will aid you as you make your changes. The negative cultural norms you will want to try to change or to avoid as you do things your own way.

Step Two. Get the Facts and Separate Fact From Fiction

There are two kinds of facts that are of interest in the Lifegain program. One involves the health information that is necessary to plan a program of change and the second involves the facts about ourselves that we will need to apply to our own lives.

The first set of facts are important because incorrect "facts" can cause unnecessary difficulties. So often when people have a health problem, they want to jump right in with a frenzy of activity. It is wise to find out the "real" facts, to separate the facts from fiction, and to understand the logic of what you are doing before you actually begin your program.

For the second set of facts, a series of analytical tests are provided so you can get objective information about yourself and your present situation, and separate these from the fiction that might exist in your mind. You analyze such things as your drinking or your exercise habits, how much stress there is in you life, what you like or dislike about smoking.

Perhaps even more importantly, you learn to separate facts from the negative judgments we sometimes make about ourselves, judgments that tend to be formed by the very same culture that got us into the bad health practices in the first place. Our culture has a very strong tendency to blame the victim rather than to help him. Thus those of us who are overweight or who smoke or who don't exercise, frequently end up calling ourselves slobs or weaklings rather than understanding the facts about ourselves and looking for a solution. This tendency we have to blame ourselves actually gets in the way of our efforts to change.

In Step Two the purpose is to look at the facts in a nonjudgmental, objective way and open-mindedly decide what is truly best to do. You don't place blame, you don't judge, you don't point fingers, because the guilt and put-downs drain us of the very energy we need for change and can even cause resistance. So you look at the facts, not as a parent or a judge placing blame, or as a child defending himself, but as an adult who has the real facts making intelligent choices, with no negative judgments to put yourself down.

We saw those forces at work in one overweight teen-age boy who had tried to lose weight in more than ten different crash diets with little success. Each time he tried, he would berate himself for past failures and end up consoling himself with large intakes of food before the new diet had barely begun.

Similarly with smoking, the smoker might say to himself, "Smoking is a stupid habit. If you had any guts you'd stop." "You aren't going to tell me what to do. I'll smoke if I want to." How much better it would be if the adult part of the person had said, "What are the consequences if I do or don't stop smoking, and what do I do to change?"

Step Three. Find and Build Supportive Environments

It is our experience that before any plan is implemented, it is critical that we create a supportive environment in which the plan has a reasonable chance of success. If this is not done, the best programs are likely to fail. If it *is* done, even the weakest programs have some chance of success.

One of the most important elements in creating this supportive environment is to build effective support groups that will help you achieve your objectives in the change programs. When the Lifegain program that you have selected is implemented in organizational settings, formal support groups are developed as an integral part of the ongoing program. When you are working this program for yourself, it will be necessary for you to develop those support groups on your own. Ideas for doing this are provided in each chapter.

In addition to the support groups, we can work on other aspects of our environment, modifying our schedules, redesigning our centers of interest, having a walk before dinner instead of cocktails.

Think if you were trying to play the guitar. It would be harder to do if your family and friends were negative. It would be easier if they encouraged you: if you played and they said "more, more;" if they asked you to play at parties; if they told you when you were getting better; if they told you they enjoyed your playing; if they chipped in to pay for lessons; if they established a family music hour every week and joined you; if they had you make a record and gave it to friends.

The same kind of support works for any of the health behaviors. You will need to look around, see what kind of support you can find, then build from there, sustaining the supportive atmosphere that helps you.

Recent research indicates an even greater importance to support groups than ever before realized, even in laboratory animals. When given electric shocks, animals caged alone will have a higher ulcer rate; if caged with litter mates, they will have a low ulcer rate.

Drs. C. B. Nuckolls and John Cassel, of the University of North Carolina, studied emotional support in pregnant women. Each woman took a Life Change Test to determine stress and another test designed to measure relationships with husband, family, and the immediate community in terms of the support she was receiving or could anticipate receiving. Ninety percent of the women with high stress scores but low support scores had one or more complications of pregnancy; only 33 percent of women with equally high stress scores but with high support scores had any complications.

Talk over your plan with your family or friends and ask for their support. Explain what you're going to do and just what will hinder or help you, so there's a better chance of their providing you with the support you will need.

Even the most individualistic of us is greatly influenced by others. Whether we recognize it or not, our need to be part of an inner circle, to feel important and near the center of things is very strong. The permission giving of our group can be good or bad for things the individual would never do otherwise. It is amazing how little permission it sometimes takes to lead a person to do things he or she might otherwise not consider.

So even if you are generally an individualist, it's important to surround yourself with some key people who really think it's okay — in fact, great — for you to get up at dawn and jog, to swim after work at the "Y," to diet, to join a health club, to not drink it you don't feel like it, to do what you want to do.

Tell them that you seriously need their help and what specific things they could do to give you emotional support. Seek out those who share your concerns. And welcome others who seek you out.

Where Lifegain workshops and support groups are available, they can be a major resource for change. Whether people are trying to exercise, lose weight, stop smoking, or feel better about themselves mentally and emotionally, they all face some of the same obstacles, and they can give each other the support they need.

One woman said the last time she tried to quit smoking on her own she would tell people, but no one around her really cared. This time, in her Lifegain support group people clapped and cheered when she announced she was in her second week of nonsmoking. "It was as though I had just won the Nobel Prize," she said. "I found it easier and easier after that."

In the group meetings, it's routine to find this kind of support. As one support group member reported, "We invite people to become friends, to bring friends into the group, to get together between and after meetings." In fact, there is a regular system for people to call each other to check on progress and give support between meetings. People in the group become so close it would be a shame not to continue the friendships. And it is these friendships that make it easy for us to maintain the changes that we make.

Step Three in each chapter will tell you where to look in your community for organized groups. Such groups will provide you at least one ready-made culture that will support and encourage your efforts. They will also confront any behavior on your part that tends to decrease your chances of success,

and the other members of the group will serve as models to show it can
be done.

Step Four. Put Your Plan Into Action

Armed with facts, aware of the influence of culture, and with a supportive
environment, you are now ready to go into action to set up your new
system.

If you have followed the first three steps systematically and well, the
fourth step will follow as a completely free choice. The objectives will be
choices of your own rather than someone else's vision of what you "should"
or "shouldn't" do. You want a plan you can believe in. You want to decide
just what level of commitment you are ready to make. Without a commitment based on your own free choice, very little will be accomplished. When
it's you own decision, you can find much more success.

The extent and openness of your commitment is also important. If you
make the commitment only to yourself, silently, it may not stick. But if
you make it to someone else, you are more likely to have the motivation
to follow it.

In each chapter we have surveyed the programs experts have put together
and have assessed them. We give you a number of alternate paths we consider
of high quality so you can choose a program that suits you. What is good for
one person is not necessarily good for another, so you are urged to design
your own plan, choosing from among the possibilities listed those most
appropriate and appealing to you, even adding strategies of your own once
you understand the basic elements of the program. You should, of course,
include whatever advice you get from your physician on your specific health
problems and needs.

There are certain key characteristics that are found in all successful plans.
They are based on facts. They allow for sustained and lifetime commitment
to the changes suggested. They emphasize having fun and enjoying yourself,
and they are compatible with the seven Lifegain steps being presented here.

For every one of the plans a major principle is to make your initial goals
easily achievable, so you can get a quick taste of success. You start out
gradually. You begin by building the proper environment first. If you're
going to lose weight, you get rid of all the fattening foods in the house, make
out a grocery list of nonfattening foods, discuss your plans with your family.
When the first steps are easy, it builds your confidence. When the environment is right, then the rest of the action plans become easier. The result — a
plan that is as customized for you as your fingerprint, so that you are happy
with it, so it will work best for you.

You actually see yourself making progress instead of playing the old game
of knowing you should do something about your health but somehow never

doing it, and ending up making a joke about it instead at the next cocktail party or moaning at the bridge club how you can't lose weight.

Also in Step Five we have included some examples of what other people have done to bypass or confront cultural norms in their lives. Here you will see how people have been able to follow nutritious diets, exercise in a no-exercise world, and keep their sights on the positive actions despite the negative norms that surround them.

Step Five. Keep Track and Tune In

In marathon running "the wall" is a distress zone of discomfort and pain that the runner reaches at about 20 miles. The runner has to get past the aches, cramping muscles, wracking lungs, and sudden loss of nerve that are so common.

Some runners distract themselves by counting numbers or imagining they are somewhere else. But the most successful runners outwit the wall by keeping in constant touch with what is happening. They respond to the feedback they get from their internal sensations, monitoring distress signals coming from their bodies, adjusting their pace, relaxing.

A similar thing can happen when you review your progress in a specific health area. You can get in touch with what is really happening by tuning in to your reactions. You tune in to your body, not judging, just listening. You tune in to how your body feels, to how it is reacting to the experience.

You tune in to how you feel when you overeat, overdrink, are tense and anxious all day; and you compare that to how you feel when you've exercised, eaten nutritiously, stayed relaxed. And as you stop smoking or start running, you tune in to how much better your body feels.

In Step Five you not only tune in but keep track of how you are doing. How much trimmer is your waist? How much better do you feel? This feedback to yourself of how well you are doing acts as a spur to further action. Some people find it helpful to keep diaries of the changes they make and how they feel about them. This kind of keeping track helps, for the problem that loomed so huge at the beginning seems more accessible when you see that you have succeeded with the first steps.

Too many programs are concerned with activities instead of results. It's not the number of meetings you attend that is important, it's the quality of results — how you're doing. It's feeling the joy and exhilaration of your total wellness.

Sometimes we need a big push in the beginning. Like a rocket, we need that initial thrust to get started, to get out of the cultural framework we're in; then we can cruise along with much smaller expenditures of energy.

Jim Bernstein, a Lifegain ex-smoker, talks about how tough not smoking was for the first few days; how now, two years later, it's nothing but a joy.

Tom Smith remembers how it was through the first ten days of jogging, its aches and pains; now if jogging is left out of his day, he feels denied.

Step Six. Reward Yourself and Have Fun

No change is going to stick unless it is rewarding to you in terms of fun, satisfaction, recognition, status, material rewards, or the enjoyment you are having with others in your program. You need to feel good about the change you are making.

It is best when the plan you have undertaken is rewarding in itself, giving you a sense of control over your life that provides a satisfying sense of achievement.

Choose activities you like the most. Vary them. Be creative with them. Hold onto the things you enjoy and make them part of your regular activities. Include social activities. Have fun. Reward yourself each time you accomplish an objective.

So often people approach health changes as if they are problems instead of possibilities for improvements. You have to change that. If you're in it for life, you have to get fun and enjoyment from it. You've got to make eating fun, exercise fun. You've got to build social relationships into the program. There will be very little advantage to living a long life if it's going to be a miserable one. It's no bargain to add five years of misery to your lifespan. It's the quality that counts.

Step Six of each chapter helps you invent and plan rewards for yourself right from the very beginning, as soon as you complete the first step toward change. And if you succeed in your plan, you *deserve* a reward.

Step Seven. Reach Out to Others

The final section of each chapter discusses how to reach out to others. Just as you need the help of others to achieve your goals, others may need help from you to achieve the goals that they have set for themselves. When you understand how the culture operates and what you can do about it, you're in a unique position to help others. You can help them in their struggles simply by giving them the support you have learned about. This is a step that can begin almost immediately by providing help to others you are working with, and you don't have to wait until you personally have accomplished your objectives.

It helps you, too. You reinforce your own behavior and are more likely to benefit from the programs and maintain your gains. Statistics indicate that those who are helping others to bring about change are the ones who are most likely to maintain it for themselves.

The reaching out section gives illustrations of what people have done to establish new patterns in their families, schools, neighborhoods, work places, and government. The Lifegain method is especially good for reaching out to help your family without being a nag.

As one girl said, "I suddenly realized it's not caring to let someone do something that is bad for them. My sister smokes a lot. I used to shrug my shoulders and call her a dummy, but figured it was her business. Now I feel with the whole family acting together and being supportive, we can help her stop smoking. It's the greatest gift any of us could give her."

But so often the way we try to keep people out of bad health habits actually pushes them into the habits. Because parents make smoking, drinking, and driving fast forbidden fruit, it makes those activities seem great. The child's reaction: "I'm going to get independence and freedom by smoking." Or perhaps the parent says, "You don't have to behave like everybody else." But it isn't that easy.

The Lifegain way is to help people understand the problem in a cultural perspective, to help them understand and learn to recognize the peer pressures, and to help them get accurate information about a problem — not just the propaganda, but the real facts.

People can take charge of their own lives. Time and time again we have seen people make significant changes in their lives with the help of others. Sometimes people need help in thinking through what is really best for them. We all need help in achieving the goals that we set for ourselves. Most people don't really want to have bad health. They want to be helped by their friends and the people who care about them.

If your husband is trying to lose weight, it would help him greatly if you didn't put sweets and starches on the table for the rest of the family. If your wife is trying to become a nonsmoker, tell her on the days she doesn't smoke how proud you are of her, or how great you think she's doing — even tell her she's sweeter smelling and nicer to kiss now.

So many families and friends don't talk about their lives at all, their dreams, their frustrations. Try talking over how you want things to be, things you want to change, what you can do together to make things better, to help each other.

One way is to give everyone an opportunity to develop one or two things he or she would like to change most to improve either mental well-being or physical health.

In family settings, let the children comment on parents as well as on themselves. Go over the list together, decide on goals, and have future meetings to see how much progress you made toward the goals. One family, the Jacksons, found these meetings so helpful they decided to establish a family tradition of having them as a regular part of their weekly schedule.

The Jacksons' discussions revealed that several of the family members were dissatisfied with communications within the family. Mostly it was the older members telling the younger members what to do and the younger members smoldering about it. The family started spending more time together talking about the things that were important to each member. The grandmother said she wanted to do more things around the house, had felt useless being waited upon by the rest of the family. The boys felt they were not learning any skills. The father, an engineer, decided to teach them electrical work and house repairs. The family all professed to wanting to develop healthy bodies, but they spent little time together in exercise activities. They decided to get a family membership in the local "Y" and spend more of their family time together participating in family recreation programs.

Another family found they were spending a great deal of time criticizing and putting each other down and very little time having fun and enjoying each other. They decided to do at least one fun thing together every day, to go for a walk or to a movie, eat out, play a game, go on a picnic, or spend some time exercising together. These ideas came from suggestions all family members made. And they make it a point now to say nice things to each other.

Have a way-you'd-like-in-your-wildest-dreams discussion. Imagine a perfect situation and environment, the life and health you want if your dreams could come true. Children may not always know what they want to do in life, but they can decide what kind of a person they want to be in terms of health, activities, and relationships with others. This exercise can help them get started on that kind of a life plan that is important no matter what the career turns out to be.

LIFEGAIN'S GUIDING PRINCIPLES

Throughout these seven steps there have been running the threads of certain guiding principles that strengthen the entire process. They are often stated, sometimes implied in the suggestions and advice proffered. To sum them up: be alert to the impact of culture; base your change effort on sound information; involve others where possible, and build a support program suited to your own individual needs; focus on results rather than on activities; reward yourself for your accomplishments; and finally, reach out to others to help them with the changes that they are trying to develop in their own lives.

Total Health

There has been a great deal of interest in recent years in a concept known as holistic health, a concept that stresses the interrelationships that exist between one health area and another, and between the many parts of ourselves. This total health principle pervades the Lifegain program.

While it is necessary to focus on one health area at a time as we try to change our practices, it is well to keep in mind this essential interrelationship.

Each of the chapters stands alone in its area, but the implications for total health are profound.

Working on any one area will have a positive impact on many others. For example, cutting out smoking will help your exercising, exercising will help you lose weight and fight stress, good nutrition will help with energy and mental health. Everything is tied together. In fact, sometimes it's almost impossible to change one health practice without changing others. Many people find it much easier to give up smoking when they also work on exercise and stress.

And the benefits don't just add up, they multiply. If you exercise, you have five times less chance of dying from heart disease as an inactive person. The odds are even greater in your favor if you are not overweight, eat properly, and are not a high-stress reacting person. Every factor raises your body that much higher to total health. And all in such a short time. Many of the programs start working in days.

THE LIFEGAIN PROGRAMS

Each of the next eight Lifegain chapters concentrates on one important area of total health — exercising, becoming a nonsmoker, becoming an intelligent eater, staying slim, handling alcohol, avoiding accidents, managing stress, getting along with yourself and others. These for most of us are the eight most important areas to consider in reaching total good health.

We recommend that you read each of the chapters, even though you may need help in only two or three areas, because you will discover a great many eye-opening things about how the culture affects us. And even if you do not need help, you will learn many ways to help others.

The first part of each chapter explores the cultural norms that underlie our current health practices and the impact they have on us and on the national health picture, in the lives they cost and in the ways they sap the quality of our everyday existence.

The second part of each chapter gives the details of the Lifegain program in that area, analyzing its importance in your own personal life, helping you to decide how you want to handle that health factor in *your* life, and suggesting ways that you — step by step — can set up an action plan for yourself.

The seven basic steps of Lifegain are integrated into each chapter so that you can follow the systematic approach that has been suggested in this chapter. The system analyzes your own situation and feelings and goals, then helps you set up your own action plan. And it starts you off with some specific first steps that you can take immediately to improve your quality of life, then follows through with long-term goals and suggestions of ways for you to support yourself emotionally and culturally as you embark upon and sustain your change.

5 How To Be Fit for Life

At 44, Harry was overweight and woefully out of shape. He could remember when he was young, fit, and vigorous. He wasn't a letterman but he used to participate in just about everything. He'd felt good then, kept his weight down, slept well, been better off all around. Well, maybe he couldn't change his age, but, by golly, he could make himself fit again. There would be no more huffing and puffing over a flight of stairs, or wheezing, coughing, and back pains over moving a refrigerator or shoveling a little snow. Harry would do something about it, starting first thing tomorrow.

Harry got up an hour earlier than usual the next day so he could get some jogging in before breakfast. He drove directly to the high school since the school track seemed the logical place to run. Unfortunately, Harry hadn't considered the fact that the athletic field was enclosed by a high chain link fence and that the gates might be locked, which they were. He decided to go back home and jog around the block. The cement sidewalk wouldn't be as soft and springy as the regular track, but he had his old tennis shoes on and figured it wouldn't be too bad.

Harry figured he'd circle the block about ten times to start with — that didn't seem like a lot when you consider how he used to run. After the first time around though, Harry was virtually staggering, and he couldn't even complete the second lap without slowing to a walk. He walked one more time around the block, tried to break into a run again, and gave it up. It was getting lighter now and he'd noticed the paperboy and two neighbors who looked at him strangely. Embarrassed and exhausted, he limped back into the house.

Harry had decided to skip lunch and take a long walk instead, but Bill, Tom, and Joe came by his office to go to lunch together as usual. When he told them he planned to take a walk instead of going right to the restaurant, they acted as though he were crazy. They told him he wasn't in any worse shape than anyone else, he should act his age, and besides, lunch wouldn't be the same without him. In the end, Harry gave in — his legs felt a little stiff anyway from the morning run.

After dinner Harry announced he was going to the local store several blocks away to get the evening paper, intending to walk there and back. But since he was going anyway, his wife asked him to pick up a few things there and drop their daughter off at her Girl Scout meeting, so Harry ended up taking the car.

When he arrived back at the house, Harry went down to the basement to look for his son's set of weights. Now that the boy was off to college, they were put away, but he finally found them. The bar had been set for 100 pounds, which didn't seem like too much. After all, his son had been lifting it, so a grown man should be able to handle that much.

The next day Harry's doctor told him that the strained back muscles would clear up in about a week, as would his bruised shins where the weights had hit him when they dropped.

WHERE HARRY WENT WRONG

Harry really had a good idea. He recognized that he was out of shape and that this was dangerous to his health. He had good intentions for doing something about it, too, but somehow everything went wrong. The worst part is that Harry can't understand what happened because he doesn't realize that much of his problem is caused by the lifestyle he shares with those close to him, a lifestyle tnat contributed to his getting out of shape in the first place and now frustrates his attempts to improve himself.

Every attempt he made to change his life brought him into conflict with the other members of his cultures at work and at home.

THE CULTURE TRAP

We live in a nonexercise culture.

How many people combed their hair this morning? How many do you think exercised their hearts by running, swimming, or bicycling for even 10 or 15 minutes? How we look seems to be more important than how our hearts are doing.

People feel deprived if they have to walk down to the mailbox, if their car isn't in the closest spot in the parking lot.

More than half the people surveyed in connection with the Lifegain program said they belonged to groups which hold negative norms about exercising.

The average family has the TV on for six or more hours a day.

Walking, one of the best forms of exercise for the heart, has all but disappeared as a regular part of people's lives. We drive now.

Of all Americans, only about one-quarter of us believe we get enough exercise. And paradoxically, people who don't exercise usually think they get enough exercise. Or they consider anything that takes exertion as work and do their best to avoid it.

The culture is changing in some groups. In them you'll find people in middle age, and even senior citizens, who are remarkably fit. They have experimented with exercise, found they love it, and love to feel fit. And they have purposely put themselves into groups that also enjoy and appreciate exercise and sports.

But many of the attempts are ineffective. A survey taken by the President's Council on Physical Fitness found, for example, that although more than 25 million adults say they run, two-thirds of them don't run often enough or long enough to gain the benefits they should from exercising. So the chances are that even if you consider yourself an active person, you may not get enough exercise, or the right kind.

It's been proven over and over that persons who lead the most sedentary lives have a mortality rate from coronary heart disease many times that of active individuals. In fact many doctors feel lack of exercise is one of the biggest risk factors in heart disease. Regular exercise not only strengthens the heart, it also affects other risk factors, often lowering cholesterol levels and decreasing high blood pressure.

"Take it easy," may be the worst advice anybody could give you.

Study after study shows the correlations between exercise and good health. One study on 3600 longshoremen over 22 years showed that a regular pattern of hard physical work sharply reduces the risk of dying from heart attacks. Men doing hard physical work had only half the risk of a fatal heart attack as the entire group of workingmen. If a man had a combination of no hard work plus heavy smoking and high blood pressure, his risk for a fatal heart attack was increased by as much as 20 times.

Other studies show people who exercise sleep better, have lower cholesterol levels, can work harder with less physical and mental fatigue, and have less desire for cigarettes, alcohol, and drugs. And many physicians involved in exercise programs say that as people progress in an exercise program such chronic conditions as ulcers, arthritis, asthma, and digestive disturbances often disappear.

So it does pay to exercise. In the following Lifegain program we tell you both the ways to find the best exercises and the ways to control the cultural aspects that work against engaging in it.

THE LIFEGAIN LIFELONG EXERCISE PROGRAM

Step One. Understand Your Own Culture

The person who really wants to commit to a change should first closely examine his or her cultures and identify those elements that will support the better behavior and those that are likely to counteract the efforts to change. At the same time the analysis will pinpoint the people who may be able to provide support for the change.

Right now think about your own groups and what their attitudes are on exercise.

Is it usual in one or more of your groups —

☐ for people to be pretty much physically inactive?

☐ for people to be primarily spectators as opposed to participants in athletic programs?

☐ for people to look at women who jog or run regularly as a bit unusual?

☐ for people to use their cars to go short distances even when there is no need to do so?

☐ for people to be surprised if someone chooses to climb stairs when an elevator or escalator is available?

☐ for people to look on exercise programs as grim and unpleasant rather than a source of enjoyment?

☐ for people to get exercise only on Saturday or Sunday and miss the rest of the week?

☐ for people to put off exercising until their weight is down, or their work load is lighter, or the children have grown up?

These are just a few of the norms that can contribute to lack of physical fitness. But remember, most of them can be changed, and you will see how to do this by taking the following steps.

Step Two. Get the Facts and Separate Fact from Fiction

A lot of misunderstandings exist about exercise and physical fitness. What do you know about exercise? Test yourself on how many of these answers you know.

Who Should Exercise?

Everyone. How and how much will depend on your condition and your age. It will help you to feel better at any age. And it doesn't take nearly as long to get in shape as it took you to get out of shape. Even for almost totally inactive people, significant improvement in fitness can occur in only a few weeks.

I'm Not Really an Athlete, What's In It for Me?

There are both physical and mental rewards. Your heart and lungs become healthier, your muscles stronger, your joints more flexible, your movements more coordinated and graceful. Your circulation improves, your skin looks better, flabbiness firms up, extra pounds drop. You feel better, sleep better, work better. Stress and tension decrease. And it's fun.

Doesn't Exercise Make You Eat More?

Moderate exercise actually curbs your appetite and helps to counteract overeating. Studies find that when people are sedentary, most of them overeat. Think of farmers who pen up animals they want to fatten.

What If You're Worried About Getting Heart Trouble?

Exercise and the resulting physical fitness can help insure against heart attack. The development of stamina actually builds up cardiovascular-respiratory endurance and is one way to reduce risk factors for coronary artery disease. A University of California study showed that young adults who exercised regularly were 14 times less likely to have a heart attack or circulatory or lung disease than those who did not exercise. In fact, vigorous physical activity, even in middle life, appears to provide significant protec tion against heart attacks. The incidence of heart attacks is 55 percent higher among middle-aged men who exercised little or not at all after their college years than among those who had regular vigorous physical activity. A study of 17,000 Harvard graduates showed almost twice as many heart attacks in those who participated in strenuous sports only three hours per week or less as compared to those who exercised more than that.

Many recovered heart attack victims have built up their endurance so much that they now run marathons. In Hawaii, Dr. Thomas Bassler reports 26 runners in the Honolulu Marathon last year were recovered heart attack victims and six had had coronary bypass operations.

What Actual Effects of Exercise Can You Measure?

In addition to such things as being able to swim farther, run farther, and score better on fitness tests, you can measure long-term changes in lung capacity and pulse. For example, with physical fitness your pulse rate is reduced. The pulse rate for a sedentary human is 80 to 90 per minute, but for an athletically trained adult it is only 55 to 60. The heart beating thousands of times less per day is much healthier, doctors say.

Does Exercise Really Relax You?

Yes. And strangely, fatigue as well as tension and insomnia often disappear from being chronic complaints when exercise becomes part of your lifestyle.

What If You Tend to Get Backaches?

Backaches are often the result of poor physical fitness. Proper exercise can often eliminate backache problems. If you have had back problems in the past, be certain to consult with your physician before beginning an exercise program.

If You Are Already Run-Down, is Exercise Really Going to Make a Difference?

Yes, exercise truly can make a difference, and the effects don't take long to happen. In just a few weeks you feel better, you look better, and you are better.

And scientific studies prove it.

At the University of Toronto, men and women over the age of 60 who began to exercise regularly were found in only seven weeks to have a level of fitness of persons 10 to 20 years younger.

At his clinic in Dallas, Dr. Kenneth H. Cooper reports that with exercise, diabetics were able to reduce medication; many exercisers said their stomach ulcers, lung ailments, and insomnia improved or disappeared completely; and subjects had less fatigue.

Even simple calisthenics help. A new German fitness program, for example, has just been designed with exercises for men and women who spend most of their time behind desks, in cars or jets, or sitting in front of a television set. They estimate a 10 percent increase in strength in one week, a 40 percent increase in three months.

A 12-month program of moderate exercise by men aged 33 to 55 at NASA resulted in the employees reporting that they could work harder both physically and mentally, they enjoyed their work more, and found their normal routine less boring. And the exercise program resulted in weight loss, decrease in food consumed, less stress and tension, increased physical activity beyond the program, expanded recreational activities, more adequate sleep and rest, and reduction in how much they smoked.

THE FACTS ABOUT YOUR PERSONAL FITNESS

If you want to improve your physical condition, you must first get the facts about your current condition, which the following tests will give you. If you haven't been examined by a physician in a long time, are over 40, or have any history of back problems, you should also consult with your physician before beginning any program of physical conditioning to make certain that the program you are starting on is OK for you. He or she might also want to recommend a special exercise program, particularly suited to your individual needs.

Remember, as you answer the questions below, you should not view them in a judgmental way. Because you are not exercising doesn't necessarily mean you're lazy. Just establish the facts without feeling guilty or defensive, so you can decide what is the next best step for you.

Do you exercise for at least 20 minutes every other day?	Yes	No
Do you check out your physical fitness level regularly using exercise tests or even when you walk up stairs or run for a bus?	Yes	No
If you are over 40, do you check out your physical fitness level with your physician at the time of your physical examination or screening?	Yes	No
Can you run for a bus or train without getting out of breath?	Yes	No
Do you feel full of energy?	Yes	No
Are you engaged in a specific physical fitness program of some sort on a regular basis, and do you get at least the equivalent exercise of walking ½ to 1½ miles four times a week?	Yes	No

Does it feel good to move your body?	Yes	No
Do you enjoy walking, dancing, digging in the garden, playing ball, other exercise activities?	Yes	No
If you are familiar with the aerobics charts for people of your age and sex, are you at least at a "good" level?	Yes	No
Do you have some way of keeping your body flexible and your muscles in good shape?	Yes	No

If you said "No" to one or more of the questions on exercise, this could be a fantastically beneficial area for you to work on. If you are doing well already, keep it up, and consider ways that you can carry your program to other people.

Even a program of just moderate exercise can help people lose weight, sleep better, have more energy, be less depressed and irritable and more relaxed in coping with problems. And you're lucky, because it's also a lot of fun.

PHYSICAL FITNESS TESTS YOU CAN DO AT HOME

Some physical fitness tests should only be done with a doctor, but the following tests can be done at home.

Taking a Pulse. Place three fingers on the artery on the thumb side of the wrist. Move around until you find it. Do not use the thumb. Or take the pulse in the neck, feeling firmly for the neck artery with your fingers on either side of the Adam's apple. Count pulse beats for six seconds timed by the second hand on a watch or clock. Add zero to get the pulse rate per minute.

Your pulse reflects your heartbeat. A healthy pulse has a good bounce and a regular rhythm. If your pulse is weak or irregular, see your doctor.

The Hoptest for Fitness. (If you are seriously overweight or have not exercised regularly, do not take this and the following tests until you complete a preconditioning program of increased activity and regular walks. In fact, why not get up right now and take a walk. Then a little later, take the test.)

First take your pulse while sitting at rest.

Then hop 25 times on one foot and 25 times on the other foot. Take your pulse immediately.

Sit for two minutes and take your pulse again.

Most people's pulse will be about 60 to 80 beats per minute before the test. If you are in good shape your pulse should not go up more than 50 points immediately after the hopping, and after a two-minute rest should be back to within 5 or 10 points of your resting pulse before the test.

If you have shortness of breath, chest discomfort, or dizziness while hopping, stop the test and check with your doctor.

The Stool/Step Test for Heart/Lung Fitness. (You should not take this test if you have heart or lung trouble, or are more than 20 percent overweight. If at any time during the test you have pain or discomfort, stop immediately.)

You need a stool or chair that is 15 to 18 inches off the floor and a watch or clock with a second hand.

First: step up and down on the stool once every ten seconds. Continue for two minutes. If your pulse is over 100, stop.

Second: step up and down another minute. (Stop if you feel pain.) At the end of the minute, wait 15 seconds, then count your pulse for the next 15 seconds. Wait another 15 seconds, and count your pulse for 15 seconds. Add the three pulse scores. The lower your score, the faster your heart was able to recover, and the healthier your heart and lungs are.

If your score was . . .	Your condition is . . .
61 to 67	Excellent
68 to 89	Good
90 to 97	Average
98 to 109	Below average
110 or above	Poor

Dr. Kenneth Cooper's 12-minute Run/walk Test. If either of the first two at home fitness tests were satisfactory, you can then check yourself further with this test. Mark a starting place. Start running. When your breath gets short, walk awhile; then run again; walk; run. Have someone time you 12 minutes using a watch with a second hand. Determine the distance you've traveled. (Either use your local high school track or on a level road mark off the miles with your car to measure the distance.)

Check your fitness against Dr. Cooper's chart.

Men Under Age 35:

Fitness Category	Distance Covered
1. Very poor	Less than 1.0 miles
2. Poor	1.0 to 1.24 miles
3. Fair	1.25 to 1.49 miles
4. Good	1.50 to 1.74 miles
5. Excellent	1.75 miles or more

For men over 35 years of age, 1.40 miles in 12 minutes is considered the Good category.

Women Age 30-39:

Fitness Category	Distance Covered
1. Very poor	.85 mile
2. Poor	.85 to 1.04 miles
3. Fair	1.05 to 1.24 miles
4. Good	1.25 to 1.54 miles
5. Excellent	1.55 miles or more

Women's Optional Three-Mile Walking Test. (No running.) Time how long it takes you to walk three miles.

Fitness Category	Time for Women
1. Very poor	51 minutes or more
2. Poor	51 to 46:31 minutes
3. Fair	46:30 to 42:01 minutes
4. Good	42:00 to 37:30 minutes
5. Excellent	Less than 37:30 minutes

Step Three. Find Or Build Yourself A Supportive Environment

There's a joke around about people who belong to Exercisers Anonymous. Whenever they get the urge to exercise they sit down and watch television until the craving goes away. This is not the group to ally yourself with!

Instead, try to form a Lifegain group or find another group specifically designed to promote physical fitness: the "Y," a health club, jogging groups, tennis clubs, hiking clubs, evening sports classes at schools or churches — all are cultures which promote physical fitness. See if you can find a friend to sign up with you; if not, you'll find new friends in the new sports group.

For the person who has difficulty finding support in the cultures he or she already belongs to, joining at least one culture where you will receive already built-in understanding and support can make a real difference. It's often very difficult for people to exercise completely on their own. But few of us would break an exercise appointment if someone were waiting for us in the park.

One group of women who worked in a factory doing detailed work helped each other by walking at lunch time as a group.

Maybe you can arrange with some friends at work to use part of your noon break for some rapid walking. Perhaps there is a hiking club in your area that you could join for Sunday afternoon hikes. Maybe a dance or swimming group is meeting at your local Y. Maybe some friends would just as soon meet you at the tennis court as in a restaurant.

The main point to remember is, if you haven't created a supportive environment, it is almost impossible to act in a sustained way on the basis of good intentions.

Step Four. Put Your Own Personal Plan Into Action

SYSTEMATIC PLANNING

If you're in poor condition, you did not get that way overnight, and you're not going to become physically fit overnight. You need a systematic, step-by-step gradual plan for improvement. Think about your ultimate goal—

what you hope to achieve eventually. Then realistically set up a series of intermediate goals so you can gradually progress to achieve this goal.

Avoid the pitfall of trying to push yourself too hard, too fast or of setting up unreasonably difficult goals. It can only lead to frustration and discouragement. On the other hand, realistic intermediate goals give a constant sense of encouragement and reinforcement as each is achieved.

And when you make your plan for exercising, avoid what you consider grim or harsh, but rather build in as much fun and enjoyment as possible. Whether it's team sports, solitary jogging, or exercising to the sound of music, make it fun rather than something you force yourself to do.

Day One. Preconditioning. Right now, put this book down and take a walk just to get the feel of it. You don't have to push yourself, just have a brisk comfortable stroll. Think of yourself as a regular exerciser, as being fit and full of vigor, and of how good it feels.

Day Two. Get Set. Call your doctor for any special precautions you should follow in an exercise program.

Take the fitness tests if you haven't already done so.

Take another conditioning walk at least as long as, preferably longer than, yesterday's.

Day Three. Choose the Right Total Exercise for You. For total health you need exercise or exercises that will strengthen your entire system by increasing the power, stamina, and strength of your heart and lungs; improve your muscle tone; and increase your body's flexibility.

No matter what exercise you choose, walking is probably a good start for it. It has the advantage of providing not only exercise but an opportunity to share your exercise with other people. Even marathon runners find walking a way of being with their friends and families. One additional advantage to walking is that it is clearly something most of us will be able to do all our lives.

Most of us could benefit by putting regular walking into our schedule — an hour of walking a week, as a minimum. You might try a half hour a day for three nonconsecutive days. Start with a five-minute slow period, then speed up to about three miles an hour, and finally slow down for the last five minutes.

Some people have done well on a walking plus calisthenics program, doing them on alternate days, a half hour each day.

Calisthenics are good for flexibility and loosening tight joints. But these do not give any general conditioning to the body and circulation. They do not strengthen the cardiovascular system by making it work beyond its usual limits.

The sports that give you the highest fitness benefits are brisk walking, jogging, running, tennis, swimming, bicycling, skating, skipping rope, and cross-country skiing. They make your heart work long enough and hard enough to increase its ability to pump oxygen throughout your body. They force you to breathe hard and break into a sweat. Sometimes called cardiovascular conditioning, cardiovascular development (CVD), circulatory conditioning, or aerobic exercise, the experts all agree this is the best kind of exercise program. And most recommend such exercise at least every other day as a best bet for "endurance insurance."

For an exercise to function as a cardiovascular exercise it must be aerobic, that is, it stresses the heart and lungs just enough to promote the use of oxygen. That's what the total exercises do. With all these sports, you can begin gradually, then progressively increase both your speed and time, always strengthening your heart and lungs and increasing your endurance.

With rope skipping, for example, volunteers at Lankenau Hospital in Philadelphia were shown to have had a 168 percent increase in endurance after jumping rope *only five minutes a day for six weeks.* Jumping rope for 10 minutes can provide the conditioning effect of 30 minutes of jogging.

So this day choose which total exercise or variety of exercises you think would be the most fun for you and which your doctor approves of for you.

Take a first step toward this exercise today: find some trails for hiking, check to see where the nearest swimming facility you could use is located, buy a jump rope, call a friend to see if he or she will jog with you.

Take another preconditioning walk, going farther if possible.

Day Four. Get Started. Start gradually on the exercise you chose.

If you decide on running, start running about half as fast as you think you can. Run this half-speed for about 200 yards or 30 seconds (less if you are in poor condition). Then walk for about the same time. Keep repeating, alternating walking and running for about 15 minutes or as long as you want to spend on it. (Don't jog or run downhill; it puts excessive strain on the knees. At first you may want to walk when you come to a downhill slope.)

Whatever you choose, start easy. Do it half as strenuously or half as long as you think you can handle.

Day Five. And Ongoing. If you don't feel sore, increase your distance or speed time. You will now begin gradually to build up your endurance and strength. Don't rush it.

You should do the total exercise of your choice at least every other day, according to exercise experts, to get the maximum benefit and feel your best. If you walk, you should cover at least two miles.

Follow this program for 30 days and you will feel miraculously better. Keep it up for all your years and you will amaze yourself at how much better you feel, even better than you thought you were at your best.

EXERCISE POINTERS FOR WHATEVER EXERCISE YOU CHOOSE

Before you start on your exercise program check your present fitness level (see Step Three), and if you are going to start a vigorous exercise or sport, anything beyond what you usually do, check with your doctor.

Set aside specific times for your exercise and sport so it does not get pushed off your schedule.

If you are in only poor or fair condition, work up gradually to strengthen the muscles, lung, and heart and improve their efficiency.

Exercise on an empty stomach, before a meal, or at least no sooner than an hour after.

Wear loose comfortable clothing that won't in any way restrain you.

Before you start each exercise session do some warming up with stretching or breathing exercises, running in place, or walking briskly for one minute.

Breathe deeply when exercising; never hold your breath.

Drink enough water, including one glass before you begin. (Don't believe the old wives' tale about not drinking when exercising. It's good to replace water loss.)

If you start a calisthenics program, just do each exercise a few times. As you gain strength and stamina each day, you can increase the number.

Check your pulse occasionally when exercising. It's good to get it up to about 120 so you know you're giving your body a workout, but it should not be over 120 five minutes after you stop. If it is, you're overextending yourself.

Stop what you are doing any time you have cramps, pain or tremor in the legs, difficulty in breathing, a pounding heart, pains in the chest, nausea, or if you simply feel worn out.

If you feel a little sore after exercising, that's only because you're using some new muscles; keep it up. But if you feel *very* sore after exercising, skip the next day and start the following day at a less strenuous level. If you're only tired, do the exercising anyway; it will often pick you up and make fatigue disappear. If you're really exhausted or ill, postpone the exercise session.

As you finish exercising, taper off slowly, or walk slowly for a few minutes. Don't stand quietly in one spot, you can become dizzy and faint.

GOOD WARMING-UP EXERCISES

Before starting any vigorous exercising or strenuous sports always do some warm-ups.

The overhead stretch. Rise on your toes, reach your arms from your side to above your head, stretch toward the ceiling.

Jumping jack. Stand at attention; jump, spreading your feet and legs outward, at the same time swing your arms out and up and clap them over your head. Jump back to the starting position. Do this 10 times.

Fencer's stretch. A good warm-up exercise for stretching the legs before tennis. Put the right foot about three feet ahead of the left, with the right knee bent and the left leg straight. Lean both hands on your bent right knee and stretch your left leg back as far as possible. At the start simply stretch and maintain your balance as long as possible. Later add a gentle rocking motion.

IF YOU JOG

Jogging is fun in an upright position; don't lean. Keep your back as straight as you can and still remain comfortable; keep your head up, don't look at your feet.

Breathe deeply with your mouth open; do not hold your breath.

If for any reason you become unusually tired or uncomfortable, slow down, walk, or stop.

Select comfortable clothes. Do not wear rubberized or plastic clothing which can cause body temperature to rise to dangerous levels and interfere with evaporation of sweat.

Wear properly fitting shoes with firm soles, good arch supports, and pliable tops, such as those made especially for distance running or walking. Avoid inexpensive, thin-soled sneakers. Wear soft, well-fitting socks.

If possible, avoid hard surfaces such as concrete and asphalt for the first few weeks. Running tracks, grass playing fields, and parks are recommended.

Don't jog during the first hour after eating, or during the middle of a hot, humid day.

Whether you jog, concentrating on style and form, or whether you just rove about the countryside with a leisurely combination of running and walking that is pleasant to you, the important thing is to enjoy yourself and keep it up.

EXERCISES YOU CAN DO ANY DAY ANY TIME

In addition to your every other day total exercise sport, you may want to practice some of these exercises at home or at work for general toning, firming, and relaxations. You can do these every day or on the days you don't do your total exercise sport.

Stand straight with your abdomen in. Raise your left arm over your head with the palm facing your body. Bounce your body to the right side six times while curving the arm over your head. Repeat with the right arm.

Sit with your feet apart, arms overhead, with the fingers interlocked and palms facing toward ceiling. Bend over and touch your hands to the toes of the right foot. Come all the way back up. Touch the hands to the left foot. Repeat several times.

Stand and put your foot and ankle up on a table or desk, keeping the leg straight. With little bounces, lower your head toward the raised leg. Do this five times, then change legs.

Sit with your back erect and extend your arms to the side. Rotate your fists and arms in little circles, back 10 times, forward 10 times, and back 10 times.

Grasp the arms of a chair and lift yourself up off the chair seat. Sit back down and relax. Repeat several times.

Sitting in your chair, straighten your legs and hold them off the floor to the count of 10.

Put your arms out, palms down. Place the back of your hands against the underside of the desk top. Try to lift the desk by pushing up for five seconds. Relax.

Stand about three feet from your desk, put your hands on the edge of the desk and do five to ten pushups.

Sit forward in a chair, legs slightly apart and feet flat on floor. Clasp your hands behind your head at the neck. Bend forward on a diagonal and try to touch your right elbow to your left knee in a bouncing motion. Relax. Repeat with the left elbow to the right knee. Do five times; work up to ten.

Sitting or standing, put your arms behind your back, clasping your hands together. Keeping your arms straight, squeeze your shoulder blades together as hard as you can and try to make your elbows touch. Hold to the count of five. Relax and wiggle your shoulders. This stretches the vertebra, takes pressure off the nerves, and relieves tension.

IF YOU'RE SITTING AND WAITING OR IN A LONG MEETING

Push your arms down against the chair arms as hard as you can to the count of ten, relax. Tighten your buttocks muscle as hard as you can one at a time, then together for a count of five each. Tighten your abdominal muscles, pulling in toward your spine. Hold to a count of five. Press your feet hard onto the floor for a count of five. Tighten the muscles of one leg, hold, then let them relax. Do the other leg. Tighten your back muscles and draw your shoulders down and back. Hold to five. Relax.

ADDITIONAL WAYS TO INCREASE YOUR FITNESS

- Walk up stairs instead of taking the escalator.
- Walk several blocks to lunch instead of going to the nearest restaurant.
- Exercise at lunch.
- Walk the dog with your kids.
- Park a block away, or at the far end of the parking lot, instead of the closest spot.
- Do all errands within two miles on foot — store, library, doctor's office, friends.

- Run in place while watching the morning news.
- Join a weekly dance class.
- Take up "belly dancing," yoga, or karate.

Step Five. Keep Track and Tune In

If you jog, keep track on your calendar of how far you go each day. If you use a bicycle, stationary or otherwise, keep track of how long you bike. If you do calisthenics, keep track of how many more sit-ups you do, or push-ups, or whatever. If you swim, count your laps every week.

Don't worry if your progress is irregular. A plateau effect often occurs, especially if you're seriously out of shape.

Keep tuned in to your body. Let it direct the pace of your exercise, and feel the exhilarating new sense of power as your body becomes more fit. You'll be impressed by how your stamina and skill increase, how your waistline decreases, and your feeling of well-being skyrockets.

Step Six. Reward Yourself and Have Fun

Rewarding yourself and having fun is no problem for people who exercise. Who ever saw a frown on the face of a bike rider on a spring day or on a tennis player who hit a winning shot?

But give yourself some other rewards too: a new warm-up suit, a vacation in the Caribbean to enjoy new swimming skills, or a zingy new tennis racket.

Step Seven. Reach Out to Others

Look around, involve your family, friends, and co-workers. You'll find an added closeness when you've worked out or played together. Why not spend some time talking with other people involved with various exercise groups, visiting their facilities, and reading about their programs?

Other things you can do:

- Learn a new sport with your family and play it together.
- Instead of a big cocktail party, give an outdoor picnic with sports built into the program.
- Take your family on a hike in the nearest forest preserve next weekend instead of watching the games on television.
- Limit the number of TV hours watched each day and buy a ping pong table for some alternate family fun.
- See if you can get the community to set up some bicycle paths or hiking

trails. Rights to abandoned railroad lines can usually be obtained without undue problems.
- Suggest the next office party be a picnic.
- Put a notice on your bulletin board at work and see if anyone wants to sign up for some specific sports: bowling league, golf tournament, jogging after work.
- Talk to your medical officer, nurse, or insurance buyer at work about the possibility of a company fitness program. Be sure to tell them how effective such programs can be in increasing employee performance, reducing absenteeism, and holding down health costs.
- Suggest that your next convention have a speaker or program on exercise and the safe practice of exercise.
- Develop a Lifegain group in the neighborhood, work place, or school.
- Encourage others who are trying to exercise with praise, recognition, or other rewards.
- Talk to town leaders about expanding recreational facilities.
- Volunteer to head an exercise group.

Remember, none of these things will work by themselves, but all of them are possible aids in your wider-based program.

SOME FINAL NOTES

Almost everyone slips sometime. If you have carefully built a supportive environment, your friends will be available when this happens to you. If not, you'll have to pick yourself up. Sometimes a stretch of bad weather — or a whole winter season — can get in the way of exercising. When this happens it is necessary to have a second line of exercises ready — things you can do indoors.

The important thing to remember is that one setback need not mean the end of your plan. This is not a crash program you are involved in, not a single-shot attempt. It has a wider cultural base, with your family and friends and groups to look to for support, and a number of different options that you can pull "out of the hat" when you need them.

6 Changing Our Smoking Culture

Whether you are a smoker or a nonsmoker, your entire life, hour by hour during every day, is likely to be permeated with smoke and smoking.

It may start when you wake up, if someone in your family has a cigarette with the first cup of coffee. Fellow travelers may smoke on the way to work. At work, some of the staff are smoking by the time the first phone rings and smoke throughout the day. Even at lunch there are ashtrays on every table.

On the way home people are relaxing with a cigarette, blowing smoke at the bus stop or in the car pool. At home there may be a cigarette before dinner, cigarettes after dinner, cigarettes with coffee, cigarettes with television or bridge.

We are enticed by cigarette advertising, which uses every psychological trick in the book, from your need for peer approval, to your need for independence, to sex appeal. We see people smoking on television. Everywhere we go we are surrounded by people smoking.

Some $422 million is spent on tobacco advertising every year. We spend more on tobacco than we do on public education. We spend more on tobacco than we do on all public charities combined. We spend more on tobacco than on all our churches. We spend more on tobacco than the total cost of Medicare. The government warns us not to smoke, yet subsidizes tobacco farmers!

In the United States about four out of every ten men smoke, and three out of every ten women. About three million men and women started smoking this year, mostly young people. In fact six million teenagers are now smokers.

The subcultures people belong to appear to influence smoking habits. The biggest smokers are those aged 35 to 44, blue collar workers, those who are divorced or separated, those who went to high school but not to college.

And as the attitudes of subcultures change, smoking patterns are changing too. Half of college graduates who once smoked are now nonsmokers. Men are smoking less. And as women express themselves and gain greater levels of freedom, more women are smoking, especially teenage girls. What a tragedy that at this very time when women are beginning to attain some of the fulfillment they are seeking, they are taking up smoking, losing on one hand what they are gaining on another.

The effects of the smoking culture on our health are devastating. As one investigator bluntly put it, "Tobacco is a hazard equal to all other hazards in life combined." "It's slow-motion suicide," said former H.E.W. Secretary Joseph Califano. "Smoking is even more dangerous than we originally believed. . . . Those who ignore the facts are whistling past the cemetery."

Three studies of 1.4 million British, United States, and Canadian citizens showed that male cigarette smokers, taken as a whole, had a 30 to 80 percent greater mortality than nonsmokers. The more cigarettes smoked and the earlier they started, the higher their death rate. *One-third* of *all* their deaths would not have occurred if cigarette smokers had the same death rates as nonsmokers.

Here are the details.

Smokers of 10 or more cigarettes per day have a death rate 40 percent higher than nonsmokers. Smokers of more than 40 cigarettes per day have a death rate 120 percent higher than nonsmokers, usually dying about eight years prematurely.

Smokers have many more times the mortality from every blood vessel disease — from heart disease, strokes, and the dangerous thinning and bulging of the artery called aortic aneurysm. One out of every four heart attacks is believed to be due to smoking. Smoking can cause spasm of coronary arteries as well as narrowing and thickening; can trigger the heart into uncontrolled muscle contractions called ventricular fibrillation, and can increase the sticking together of blood platelets, making it more likely for clots to form.

Smokers have up to 20 times more chronic bronchopulmonary disease including emphysema and bronchitis.

Smokers consistently have more symptoms of cough, phlegm, wheezing, and shortness of breath than nonsmokers.

The risk of death from lung cancer, the number one cancer killer, is 20 times greater in two-pack-a-day smokers. Once lung cancer is diagnosed, in most cases it is already too late and nothing can be done. Some 80 percent of lung cancer could be *prevented*, says the American Cancer Society, if cigarette smoking were eliminated, and that would reduce the overall incidence of cancer by 50 percent! A sad fact — due to women's increased smoking — is that the death rate from lung cancer in women has more than doubled since 1965.

Smoking plays a major role in causing cancer of the larynx, mouth, throat, esophagus, stomach, intestines, bladder, pancreas, and kidney. (Eight cancer-causing chemicals have been found in cigarette smoke so far.)

Men who smoke have 100 percent more peptic ulcers; women 50 percent more.

For women on birth control pills, cigarette smoking greatly multiplies the risks of stroke, pulmonary embolism, and heart attack.

Pregnant women who smoke have twice the number of premature babies, more low birthweight babies, more miscarriages, three times more stillborns, and more deaths after delivery. In fact, scientists say one out of five unsuccessful pregnancies would have been successful if the mother had not been a regular smoker. (Even smoking by fathers when the mother is pregnant increases the rate of stillbirths.)

The smoking of parents can affect their children in many ways. More children smoke when their parents smoke; death rates in infants up to one year are one-third higher; children whose parents smoke have twice as many colds and more frequent asthma and allergies; and there appears to be a statistical correlation between smoking and sudden infant crib deaths. And did you know nicotine of smoking mothers appears in breast milk?

Total cost in medical and hospital bills and lost wages due to smoking is estimated at a shocking $18 *billion*. Cost of lost productivity to industry because of smoking-related illnesses is estimated at another $12 to 18 billion.

THE SMOKE-CULTURE TRAP

All of these problems are deeply rooted in the culture and if we are going to get a solution to them, that solution must also come from the culture — not just the solution to the individual smoker but efforts to help people to shift and change the culture itself, not just for one's own interest but for the whole society's interest.

If we see the problem in a cultural perspective, then the solution can make use of our cultural understanding. Our current approaches are obviously not doing enough. (Some 55 million people still smoke, or they stopped smoking then began again.)

One would have thought that putting the surgeon general's statement "dangerous to your health" on cigarette packages and ads would have stopped people from smoking, that the No-Smoking Days, the posters, the Kiss-me-I-don't-smoke buttons, the final messages from celebrities dying of lung cancer, the advertisements on television warning of dangers, would have made people stop. But the record shows that smoking continues to be one of our greatest health hazards anyway.

When smokers are confronted with the evidence, some few may change their behavior, but most will simply block the evidence from their deeper consciousness — it's much easier. They may decide the studies are invalid because their grandfather smoked and lived to be 80, or they may decide they would rather live a short "happy" life with cigarettes than a long life without them. The more they get committed to their decision, the more they may resist the evidence because, as one psychologist points out, to change now would be to admit, perhaps, they were wrong before.

Four out of five cigarette smokers surveyed say they would like to stop smoking if they thought they could. Many have trouble stopping because of nicotine, which has addictive powers. The strength of this addiction varies from person to person, but all smokers feel it to some extent and for many it is a powerful compelling need. Nicotine has been shown to actually stimulate nerve cells and increase heart rate and respiration, and this stimulation is one of the things smokers become dependent on. And many people have difficulty stopping because of the pleasure they derive, especially the relaxation they have learned to find.

Many say they smoke mostly because of simple habit. They have come to associate many routine events during the day with a cigarette, and when any of these events occur (a cup of coffee, a telephone call, driving the car), they automatically light up without thinking. It just seems the accepted thing to do. They may even smoke several cigarettes consecutively without ever noticing that they have smoked.

There are many reasons why people continue to smoke — the enjoyment in handling the cigarette, feeling the warmth of deeply inhaling, the relief of tension, the chemical lift of the nicotine.

What causes a person to *start* smoking? Certainly not pleasure. Anyone who has ever tried smoking remembers well their initial encounter — eyes that burn and water, coughing, choking, feeling sick and dizzy. You certainly don't feel pleasure any more than you do the first time you drink a martini. It's the same with most bad habits. We begin with something very negative, then we learn it makes us more a part of the group and we begin to say it feels nice. The unhappy initial response of most people to a cigarette is counterbalanced by its symbolism as a mark of freedom and independence, a step to adulthood.

The most important factor in a person's starting to smoke is almost always social pressure. Teenagers feel it most; usually they start smoking because of it. They are made to feel that anyone who doesn't smoke is a square, out of it. The pressure continues all through our lives, although later it may be more subtle. You may not even notice the everyday pressures until you try to give up cigarettes.

One reason so many people fail in their attempts to become nonsmokers is that they don't take all these factors into consideration. They may modify their personal habits and even deal with the problem of addiction, but they are still surrounded by the smoking culture, the seductive advertising; and the lure of smoking soon exerts its influence again. They haven't planned ahead and made conscious decisions about not going along with the seduction.

Once a new perspective is adopted, nonsmoking becomes not a sacrificial act of giving up something, but a positive act of freeing yourself of something worthless and damaging. It is a happy decision of beating an enemy that was capable of stealing your health, taking your life, and destroying the security of your family.

Some of our people say the very act of quitting gives them a new freedom and a new command not just over smoking but over their entire lives.

The people who have quit know the frightening effects of cigarette smoking on death rates from dread killer diseases.

And they learned things they didn't realize before: that cigarettes can also decrease visual perception; increase serum cholesterol and triglycerides; aggravate hay fever and asthma; decrease sex drive and response; cause skin to wrinkle years beyond one's chronological age; increase blood pressure; and aggravate gingivitis, tooth loss, and pyorrhea.

But their satisfaction with becoming nonsmokers goes beyond these devastating statistics to the quality of life. As one happy new nonsmoker said, "You remember the way you felt in the morning, how much you coughed, the stains on your teeth and hands, the cigarette smell, the holes in your clothes, the frequent colds and sinus trouble, how tired you got, the days you lost from work, being short of breath from just going up steps, the quality of your love life. It's all different now.

"In addition to years being added to your life, the quality of everyday life is improved when you become a nonsmoker. You find your cough gone, your sense of taste and smell improved, your circulation improved, and your complexion looking better. And because of increased circulation to the pelvic region, sex enjoyment increases. Any chronic bronchitis, emphysema, hay fever, asthma, and even snoring improves almost overnight."

People must decide for themselves how important the financial costs are, whether they would prefer to spend money for cigarettes or for something else. They must decide about the effect of their smoking on their children, their partner, the general community.

Note: Even if you have smoked more than a pack a day for 25 years, your risk of death is substantially reduced if you stop smoking. The longer the discontinuance, the greater the reduction in the risk. If you are a light or moderate smoker and you stay off cigarettes for 10 years, your risk of death from lung cancer and heart disease returns to that of a person who has never smoked.

THE LIFEGAIN PROGRAM TO STOP SMOKING

Step One. Understand Your Own Culture

There are many cultures that can influence a person's smoking: the culture at home, at school, the group at work, the car pool group, lunch group, neighbors and friends.

Persons may smoke because someone they admire smokes. Smoking is extolled in advertising. All the smokers on the billboards and in the magazine ads seem to be beautiful people. Most long-time nonsmokers block out the appeal of cigarette ads; the ads simply don't register. But to the person who smokes or who just recently quit, they are a strong persuasive force. For most of us who are trying to break the smoking habit, our efforts are made more difficult when we come in contact with other people who are smoking. Our family may be urging us not to smoke, but other groups and the advertising culture may be a strong influence in the other direction.

As one Lifegain participant said: "If I could stay home, I wouldn't have trouble with smoking. . . . . It's when I walk out the door and run into other people and the association with their smoking."

Only when a person recognizes how much the culture he lives in has to do with his problem can he deal with it adequately. You learn to identify the cultural influences that are affecting you. There's a click in your brain. You turn off the cultural influence and instead make your own rational, sensible decision.

Some of the norms come from the attitudes of people you come into contact with.

Think about your own business and social groups. Which of the following are norms in any of your groups?

☐ for it to be the rule to always have ashtrays on the table in restaurants and homes.

☐ for people to smoke in public buildings or restaurants.

☐ for people to think it's okay to smoke; it's nobody's business but their own.

☐ for people to automatically offer cigarettes to others.

☐ for people to smoke in closed rooms or cars when other people are present.

☐ for restaurants and bars you patronize to give matches for mementos.

☐ for young people to smoke because it is the thing to do or because they are encouraged by their friends.

☐ for people to have a smoke at intermission time at a play.

☐ for people to smoke without asking others present if it is all right.

☐ for cigarette machines to be in public places.

☐ for people not to mention it if someone else's smoking bothers them.

☐ for cigarettes to be sold next to the cash register in stores, the most important point-of-purchase position.

☐ for smoking to be presented as a desirable behavior in newspaper and magazine ads.

☐ for people not to believe or pay much attention to the warning signals that they read regarding smoking.

☐ for people to make excuses for continuing to smoke.

☐ for people to feel that the odds are in their favor that they will not die as a result of smoking.

☐ for people to give little support to others when they are trying to stop smoking.

All of these norms and attitudes could contribute to a person's smoking habit. But if you are aware of the fact that they are attitudes being imposed on you, you can liberate yourself and control them.

Step Two. Get the Facts and Separate Fact From Fiction

There are really two kinds of facts: the facts rather than the usual myths and rumors about smoking, and the facts you need to know about yourself.

First check your general knowledge. Mark these statements true or false.

- ☐ Smoking is not nearly as dangerous as the authorities say.
- ☐ Smoking is not a problem as long as the smoker feels healthy.
- ☐ If a person has smoked for years, it won't do any good to quit now.
- ☐ If a person smokes a low tar cigarette, it's okay.
- ☐ If a person has smoked for a long time, it is almost impossible to quit.
- ☐ Smoking makes it a lot easier to get through life's problems.
- ☐ Smoking doesn't hurt if you don't inhale.
- ☐ Smoking makes a person seem sophisticated, worldly, and grown up.
- ☐ Smoking doesn't hurt anybody except the smoker so it's nobody else's business.

Did you mark any of them true? If so, you are wrong. Every statement is false.

Now let's go on with questions about you.

WHY DO YOU SMOKE?

Why do you do it? Here's a test to help you think it through.

Circle the number under the word which best describes your response to the statement.

	Always/ Frequently	Occasionally	Seldom/ Never
I smoke cigarettes in order to keep myself from slowing down.	3	2	1
Handling a cigarette is part of the enjoyment of smoking it.	3	2	1
Smoking cigarettes is pleasant and relaxing.	3	2	1
I light up a cigarette when I feel angry about something.	3	2	1
When I have run out of cigarettes I find it almost unbearable until I can get more.	3	2	1
I smoke cigarettes automatically without even being aware of it.	3	2	1
I smoke cigarettes to stimulate me, to perk myself up.	3	2	1
Part of the enjoyment of smoking a cigarette comes from the steps I take to light up.	3	2	1
I find cigarettes pleasurable.	3	2	1

	Always/ Frequently	Occasionally	Seldom/ Never
When I feel uncomfortable or up-set about something, I light up a cigarette.	3	2	1
I am very much aware of the fact when I am not smoking a cigarette.	3	2	1
I light up a cigarette without realizing I still have one burn-ing in the ashtray.	3	2	1
I smoke cigarettes to give me a "lift."	3	2	1
When I smoke a cigarette, part of the enjoyment is watching the smoke as I exhale.	3	2	1
I want a cigarette most when I am comfortable and relaxed.	3	2	1
When I feel "blue" or want to take my mind off cares and worries, I smoke a cigarette.	3	2	1
I get a real gnawing hunger for a cigarette when I haven't smoked for a while.	3	2	1
I've found a cigarette in my mouth and didn't remember putting it there.	3	2	1
I smoke because my friends do.	3	2	1
I smoke because I am afraid people will make fun of me or consider me a square if I don't.	3	2	1
I smoke because I think it makes me sexually attractive.	3	2	1
I smoke because I think it's cool and sophisticated.	3	2	1

Study your answers with the highest scores to learn some of the reasons behind your smoking.

Step Three. Find or Build Yourself a Supportive Environment

You may want to find an organized group, one that follows the Lifegain plan or another plan. There are many approaches to becoming a nonsmoker and many groups available in most communities.

With or without formal programs it is usually necessary to do what we can to make our everyday environment more supportive of our new nonsmoking commitment.

One of the things that we can do to improve our environment around the issue of smoking is to keep away from those places where people are most likely to smoke. Stay away from bars and smoking sections of trains and planes. Some people have gotten rid of their ashtrays and set up their own "no smoking" areas in their houses and work places. One successful non-smoker forced himself to go outside the house before he would smoke a cigarette. This became so inconvenient he found it easier to stop.

You can establish support for yourself by finding another person to work with or even bet with.

One member of a health support group asked that she be called every evening to inquire how she had done that day. The understanding that the call was coming helped her to maintain her resolution and the inconvenience of receiving such calls eventually helped her to stop.

Often it's helpful to substitute new and more healthful addictions, such as exercising or meditating, for the old addiction. Finding some people to involve yourself with in this new activity can make it even more attractive.

This is particularly important at the beginning of a nonsmoking effort when the most help will be required. Cigarette advertisements may have a high attraction during the initial withdrawal period. In six months you will probably pay no attention to them. Ex-smokers who would like to recall how strong this influence can be, can try looking at ads from their old perspective. Be careful, though, for they could quickly bring you back in their sphere of influence! As one ex-smoker said when he tried this experiment, "I see now that when I stopped smoking, all I saw in the Marlboro ads was the strong, masculine rancher where before that the cigarettes and masculinity were inextricably intertwined."

One doctor friend of ours gives out toothbrushes and suggests that people can improve their dental future as well as their lung future by substituting the toothbrush for the cigarette. It is a reflection of our culture that using a toothbrush looks strange, while using a cancer-producing item like a cigarette seems natural. While most of us don't have the nerve to do this, some kind of oral gratification is usually helpful.

DO YOU WANT TO CHANGE YOUR SMOKING HABITS?

To test your real attitude toward smoking and to see how many things you believe that will help motivate you, take this test. Score the statements that most accurately describe how you feel.

	Completely Agree	Somewhat Agree	Somewhat Disagree	Completely Disagree
If I quit smoking I would feel better and have more energy.	3	2	1	0
Cigarette smoking might give me a serious illness.	3	2	1	0

	Completely Agree	Somewhat Agree	Somewhat Disagree	Completely Disagree
My cigarette smoking sets a bad example for others.	3	2	1	0
I find cigarette smoking to be a messy habit.	3	2	1	0
Controlling my cigarette smoking is a challenge to me.	3	2	1	0
Smoking causes shortness of breath.	3	2	1	0
If I quit smoking cigarettes, it might influence others to stop.	3	2	1	0
Cigarettes cause damage to clothing and other personal property.	3	2	1	0
Quitting smoking would show that I have willpower.	3	2	1	0
I am concerned that cigarette smoking may have a harmful effect on my health.	3	2	1	0
My cigarette smoking influences others close to me to take up or continue smoking.	3	2	1	0
If I quit smoking, my sense of taste and smell would improve.	3	2	1	0
I do not like the idea of feeling dependent on smoking.	3	2	1	0
I definitely want to be able to say next year at this time that I am a nonsmoker.	3	2	1	0

Study your answers with the highest score to see what motivational factors about smoking might be strongest with you as you begin your attempt to stop smoking.

MAKING THE DECISION

You now have some of the most important facts. It is your health and your decision. Put a check mark next to your decision.

☐   I wish to smoke at the same rate as I do now.

☐   I wish to limit my smoking to one or two cigarettes, cigars, or pipefuls a day.

☐   I wish to be a nonsmoker.

☐   I have made my commitment openly to others.

If you wish to be a nonsmoker, determine your personal plan of change. Even if you already are a nonsmoker, you might like to read through some of the material that follows to mark any techniques that would perhaps be helpful to you in reaching out to others that you'd like to help become nonsmokers.

WHEN AND HOW TO GET STARTED

Choose a specific day to begin your program, making sure you have completed the previous four steps first. Today can be the beginning — right now. Or tomorrow. Or the near future. But make it a specific time and mark it on your calendar. Try to find someone else who wants to quit and plan to help each other.

There are literally hundreds of different programs for stopping smoking, all with advantages and disadvantages. Most of them will work if you have sufficient commitment and have created an environment that will be supportive of the change. Two possible plans that people have found useful are listed below. In selecting or designing your plan make sure it fits your particular needs.

Plan A. The 10-Day Plan to Quit Cold Turkey

Day One. Increase your smoking. Force yourself to smoke as many cigarettes as you can. At least double the number of cigarettes you smoke. (Skip this step if you have cardiovascular or lung disease.)

At night when you go to bed repeat your decision several times: "Today I have chosen to stop smoking."

Day Two. Your body is in revolt against yesterday's oversaturation. Stopping will be a relief.

Get up earlier to have time for a relaxing shower or bath and a good breakfast of fruit or eggs (no sweets, no coffee).

Take a high potency vitamin and mineral tablet, plus 1000 mg. of vitamin C and a combination vitamin B complex tablet. These are to replace the vitamins in your body that have been destroyed by nicotine and to counteract stress.

As you start the day say, "I have chosen not to smoke." Repeat this every time you have an urge to smoke.

Throw away all your cigarettes immediately. Give away your lighter and matches. Put away all ashtrays in your home and office.

Eliminate all alcohol today, as well as caffeine drinks like coffee, tea, and colas, spicy foods and cakes, pies, cookies, and candy. (They are stimulants that trigger a craving for tobacco.)

Stay away from friends who smoke, and stay out of heavy smoke areas. If you go out, ask for the no-smoking section of the theater or restaurant.

Keep plenty of protein and salad snack foods around to nibble on throughout the day: fruit, celery, carrots, nuts, nonsugar chewing gum.

Drink huge amounts of water and juices. This is to flush the nicotine out of your system as quickly as possible. Drink water or juice *every hour* all through the day.

Do deep abdominal breathing when you crave a cigarette, filling your abdomen, not your chest. Sometimes the craving will go away in minutes.

Take a walk after lunch and dinner or other times you become fidgety.

When someone offers you a cigarette, say, "No, I have chosen to stop smoking."

Call the person you have chosen as a partner in the afternoon and in the evening to give each other encouragement.

Put a big jar on your dresser or desk and in it put the money you would have spent for cigarettes over the next 10 days.

Days Three Through Ten. Congratulate yourself for making it through one entire day without a cigarette. You've proved you can do it. (And if you didn't make it, don't give up or feel guilty; you've certainly made some progress and can go even further today.)

During this period you may feel irritable or tense or even have some physical symptoms. Know that they are only temporary and at the end of 10 days or sooner you will feel absolutely terrific.

Eat a full breakfast in the morning, including some protein and fruit.

Continue drinking a lot of water and juices. You can gradually add small amounts of caffeine and alcohol, but no more than two glasses or cups a day during this period.

Continue frequent snacking. (But remember to keep away from sweets.)

Continue the vitamin-mineral program.

Continue abdominal breathing when you feel the need for a cigarette.

Continue staying out of smoking areas.

Keep in touch with your partner at least once every day.

Get extra sleep at night to help you counteract the irritability you may feel during the day.

Increase your physical activity — ping pong, tennis, golf, sex — whatever will help you ward off tension.

At the end of 10 days reward yourself by spending the money you set aside in the jar.

Plan B. The Ease-Off Plan if You Want to Quit Gradually

Day One. Chart your smoking habits by making a record of every cigarette you smoke, the time you smoke it, and under what circumstances. Rate which ones you need the most with two plus signs, the ones you need the least with a minus sign, the in-between ones with one plus.

FIGURE 1. Daily Cigarette Count

Instructions: Wrap this "Daily Cigarette Count" around your pack of cigarettes and hold it fast with two rubber bands. Complete the information below if you smoke from your pack or smoke a cigarette of someone else.

Day of Week:_____ Date:_____ Pack Number of the Day:_____

Cigarette Number (Circle)	Time of the Day	Activity	Rate your Need (++,+, or -)
1			
2			
3			
4			
5			
6			
7			
8			
9			
10			
11			
12			
13			
14			
15			
16			
17			
18			
19			
20			

Adapted from: *Daily Cigarette Count,* U.S. Department of Health, Education and Welfare.

If you like to bet, find someone to make a bet with, preferably for high stakes, say $100, that at the end of the month you will have established yourself as a nonsmoker. If you can't find someone who cares enough to make the bet, make it with yourself. You care more than anybody.

Day Two. Eliminate the cigarettes you need the least, the ones marked with a minus sign.

Day Three. Continue to not smoke the "least-needed" cigarettes, but allow yourself to smoke the other cigarettes on your chart.

Begin your nutritional support program: hold coffee and colas down to two cups or glasses a day; keep alcohol down to no more than two drinks per day. Drink plenty of fluids. Eat a protein or fruit breakfast. Snack on proteins and fruits (not sweets) frequently during the day. Some experts also suggest a vitamin and mineral program with one high potency vitamin-mineral tablet every day, plus an extra 1000 mg. of vitamin C and a tablet of mixed vitamin Bs. (Vitamin Bs must be in balance with each other to work properly.)

Days Four and Five. Eliminate half of your "in-between" cigarettes, the ones marked "plus" that don't seem as important as others.

Continue your nutritional support program of low caffeine and alcohol, heavy fluids, frequent protein and fruit snacks, and the vitamins and minerals.

Begin abdominal breathing exercises, doing them every morning and evening and whenever you have difficulty keeping away from a cigarette that's not allowed.

Days Six and Seven. Eliminate the rest of the "in-between" cigarettes. You now are smoking only those cigarettes marked with a double plus.

Continue your nutritional support program and your vitamin-mineral program.

Continue your abdominal breathing whenever you need it.

Begin an exercise program to help overcome periods of stress and irritability. Do it regularly as much as you can, especially when you feel the tension building. Tennis, sex, a walk around the block, or running in place in the office can do wonders. Running has proved especially beneficial to many in smoking programs.

Days Eight Through Ten. Now you are going to start cutting down the cigarettes that are most important to you. For these three days, go ahead and smoke at those times marked with a double plus, but only smoke one-half of each cigarette. You cannot smoke any of the "less-needed" cigarettes that you eliminated previously.

Continue your nutritional support program and your vitamins and minerals.

Continue abdominal breathing as needed.

Continue exercising, concentrating on the times you feel tension.

Be sure you now start getting extra sleep at night, or even taking a nap in the daytime, so that you are well rested and can more easily remain in control all day.

It's now time to stay away from friends who smoke and to stay out of public places where smoking is heavy. Ask for the no-smoking sections of airplanes, trains, restaurants, movie theaters.

Days Eleven Through Nineteen. Every day cut one of the half-cigarettes that you are still smoking. In the morning look at the chart and decide which one it's going to be. Keep the chart with you, or copy down the times allowed on a card and carry it with you so that you absolutely will not smoke any cigarettes except for those half-cigarettes still allowed. You're now almost there. Keep telling yourself how much better and sexier you are soon going to be feeling, and think about the more than $5,000 you'll be saving in the next 10 years as a healthy nonsmoker.

Continue your nutritional support program, vitamins, and minerals.

Continue abdominal breathing as needed.

Continue exercising as needed.

Continue to get plenty of rest.

Continue to stay in nonsmoking areas so that you're surrounded by a supportive environment.

Day Twenty. This is your final quitting day. You will give up that last half-cigarette on your chart.

Continue all your support measures, especially concentrating on abdominal breathing and exercising today and for the next 10 days.

Keep nuts, nonsugar chewing gum, snack things by your side at all times.

Try brushing your teeth, using mouthwash, or sucking cough drops at the times you very much want a cigarette.

Do something special today to break your routine and reward yourself.

You may have withdrawal symptoms when you quit. In the first 48 hours especially, you may have shortness of breath, tightness in the chest, visual disturbances, sweating, headaches, gastrointestinal complaints. You may be shaky, irritable or depressed, drowsy, have insomnia, or have trouble concentrating. This is because your body is actively readjusting to the nonsmoking state. These symptoms will all pass within a few days.

Keep reminding yourself that if you can get through the next 72 hours, one hour at a time, you should be okay because the first 72 hours without any cigarettes are the worst. But Dr. Harold James, surgeon of St. Helena Hospital in Deer Park, California, says the period of craving a cigarette lasts for only about three and one-half minutes at a time, and the cravings come in cycles, sometimes several times a day, sometimes at first several times an hour. *If you can distract or reward yourself for just those three and one-half minutes* with food, a drink, a shower, exercise, a phone call, madly doodling — anything — it will get you past the craving. You can even sit and watch the second hand on your watch. Simply get your mind off cigarettes for the duration of the craving. Gradually, the periods of craving should diminish and eventually disappear.

Day Thirty. Collect on your bet. Go out and splurge it on something super. You earned it.

Step Five. Keep Track and Tune In

Whether you follow Plan A, Plan B, or any other plan, keep track of your progress.

On Plan A, since you're quitting cold turkey, your record keeping will be simple. On a regular calendar, shade in each day that you go without a cigarette with a bright orange or red marker pen. Or draw a smiling face on each day. The march of progress across the calendar will impress you.

If you follow Plan B, doing it more gradually, keep track of the number of cigarettes you have each day and mark that number on the calendar that night. You'll see those numbers go down progressively, and impressively, to zero. Even if you backslide a few days, you will be able to see the overall progress.

And tune in to see how much better you feel, how many bothersome symptoms have already changed. Think of the improvements: not so much huffing and puffing from shortness of breath and lack of stamina; better circulation and maybe better sex; no more bad breath and yellow teeth; less risk of heart disease, high blood pressure, cancer, and lung disease. When you read these advantages, they sound a little like the benefits claimed for a snake oil remedy, but they really do occur.

And feel the sense of power you have at controlling your life.

Step Six. Reward Yourself and Have Fun

You've saved a lot of money becoming a nonsmoker. In fact, if you smoke two packs of cigarettes a day for the next 10 years, you will have spent about $5,000 on cigarettes. For what you would spend in a lifetime, you could buy a yacht or a vacation house in the woods or take a year's trip around the world.

So at the end of every month from now on give yourself a special treat for still not smoking, knowing that this particular new shirt or dinner out or concert is the direct result of your having become a nonsmoker.

And since you will be feeling so much better, you are bound to be enjoying yourself more too. Try out those already healthier lungs on your favorite sport and enjoy your increased stamina. Enjoy the taste of good, nutritious food again.

Be firm with your friends (friends?) who try to get you to start again. Tell them you are feeling so much better, your food tastes so much better, and your wife, husband, boyfriend, girlfriend is so much happier, that you wouldn't think of going back to the habit. (You can smile knowingly, because only you will know whether this means you no longer smell like stale cigarette smoke or your sex performance and enjoyment have been enhanced.)

People who are members of Lifegain support groups receive great applause and support from their fellow members. One recipient of such praise said, "When I reported to the group my second week of tobacco abstinence, I felt almost as if I had just swum the English Channel." This same person reported about her earlier but not long-lasting efforts to stop smoking: "Either they never knew it occurred or my statement that I had stopped was greeted by such noncommittal comments as, 'Is that so? Isn't that nice?'"

Step Seven. Reach Out to Others

A CULTURE CHANGE PROGRAM FOR BOTH SMOKERS AND NONSMOKERS

Whether you are a smoker or nonsmoker, whether you have or haven't changed your own pattern, you can help others to change. There are a number of ways of doing this and they range from active support to open confrontation.

Encourage others not to smoke. Let them know about some of the facts you have learned in this chapter and about some of the techniques that have helped other people. If you have close friends and relatives who use birth control pills, check to see if they have read the package insert that comes with the pills warning of the sharply increased risk of heart attack and stroke for those who take the pill and also smoke.

When someone talks about the deep craving, mention, "It's interesting that the craving is supposed to last only three and one-half minutes. Have you noticed that your craving decreases then?" Remember, the trick is not to place blame, and not to be self-righteous. You can help the most by being genuinely concerned and giving positive reinforcement when a person is trying to change his or her smoking behavior.

Have you tried to help your children to think through the problems of smoking? Most teenagers who smoke start at age 13 or 14, so preventive measures should begin well *before* high school. Talk with your children about the fact that carbon monoxide has been shown to have detrimental effects on learning and about the kinds of things you all might do to reward and support nonsmoking in your family. Something to discuss: A survey shows most teenagers feel the smokers of early teens smoke mainly to show off, but that teenage girls smoke more as a rebellion against authority. Nearly all agree peer opinion is the dominant influence. The chief reasons given for success in quitting: the feeling of being in control of one's life, a sense of physical well-being, the end of cigarette bad breath and smell, and money saved.

Perhaps you could go to your local elementary school, high school, or college and try to get them to carry out a program that would help students look at smoking in a healthier perspective. The American Lung Association has a film for kindergarten through third grade, "Octopuff in Kumquat," which features children who successfully overcame a smoking octopus and created a clean air community for nonsmokers.

At many high schools, pupils are doing experiments showing the harm smoking inflicts on their bodies. The New Hampshire Lung Association, using federal funds, supplies high schools with equipment to monitor heart rate, skin temperature, carbon monoxide in the blood stream, and nervousness. The tests actually show the pupils how heart rate and carbon monoxide in the blood increase while steadiness and skin temperature decrease.

Some schools are using the Lifegain program. One sixth grade class managed to cut down on the expected percentage of new smokers by helping the students become more aware of the cultural influences being foisted upon them.

One high school teacher said these programs affect parents as well as students. "We have had many parents and students quit smoking together. Parents have called to say they have stopped smoking because the kids go home and torment them."

And once the peer pressure is against smoking, the amount of smoking in an entire school population will quickly drop. At Princeton University, for example, the percentage of smokers among students has declined dramatically from 45 percent eight years ago to 6.9 percent now, university officials say, because student peer pressure was firmly against the tobacco habit.

There are methods to reach out and influence the culture in other ways too.*

Does your company ensure that nonsmokers have smoke-free areas in which to work?

Does your hospital ban smoking and give literature to new mothers in the maternity ward on the dangers of smoking?

Does your community have — and enforce — laws against smoking in public places such as libraries, museums, movies, restaurants, elevators?

Do you have a club or professional group that can write to your congresspersons encouraging them to help eliminate government support of tobacco use?

*Excellent lists of source materials for educational materials of all kinds can be obtained from *The Smoking Digest* and in *Cancer Education Materials for the General Public,* both available from the National Cancer Institute, Bethesda, Maryland 20014.

Be sure as you talk to people about programs of change that you really involve other people and try to find "win-win," rather than win-lose, approaches.

PROGRESS IS BEING MADE

There are some cracks beginning to form in the culture walls already. About 65 percent of adults are now nonsmokers. More than 80 percent of doctors who smoked have quit. Pathologists, the doctors who look at lung cancer slides all day, have almost all quit.

And antismoking sentiment may be toughening. The latest Gallup poll shows the following:

Two Americans in three favor special areas for smokers in public places, while another 16 percent favor a total prohibition on smoking in these places — which could include trains, buses, airplanes, restaurants, and offices. Only 10 percent favor no restrictions at all.

About one-third (36 percent) of the public favors a ban on cigarette advertising.

Although smokers themselves are less inclined to take a hard line on cigarettes, there is a surprising support even among them for tougher restrictions.

Two out of every three cigarette smokers say they would like to quit.

Approaching the problem on many levels and from many angles seems to be making a difference. The change process would be speeded up even more if a systematic, culture-based approach would be taken.

LEGISLATIVE CHANGES THAT ARE STILL NEEDED

One way of reaching out is to actively participate as citizens.

The National Commission on Smoking and Public Policy, an independent commission set up by the American Cancer Society, recommends the following legislative changes:

- A phase-out over a 10-year period of the present tobacco price support system.
- Elimination of cigarettes from the Food for Peace Program.
- Reduction of insurance rates for nonsmokers.
- A ban on the sale of cigarettes to minors that is strictly enforced.
- An end to the sale of tax-free cigarettes in Defense Department establishments.
- Prohibition by state and local governments of smoking in most public

places and promotion of the separation of smokers and nonsmokers in such places as restaurants, trains, and buses.
- The banning of smoking in public schools by either students or teachers.

It's encouraging to note that even some smokers are now supporting the rights of nonsmokers.

THE RIGHTS OF NONSMOKERS

A large quantity of evidence continues to turn up on the harmful effects of tobacco smoke on innocent bystanders, such as the fact that the carbon monoxide level in a nonsmoker's blood will increase in a smoke-filled room nearly the same amount as that of the cigarette smoker. Because of this, the rights of nonsmokers are being more and more respected; many states and the District of Columbia have now passed laws that forbid smoking in various public places. In some states now, such as Minnesota and New York, smoking is forbidden in *all* public places.

How to let your opinions be known? You could wear a "Yes-I-mind-if-you-smoke" button, but one that says "Thank you for not smoking" will probably be more effective without arousing antagonism. Another Lifegain approach: If someone asks if they may smoke, give them a pleasant smile and say, "Thank you so much for asking — I really appreciate it if you do not smoke."

Sometimes more assertive techniques are necessary. If someone lights up in a no-smoking area, feel free to report it nicely to the stewardess or the manager and ask them to remedy the situation.

If smoking at work is an irritant, you can usually talk it over with your employer and work out satisfactory arrangements. But again, being assertive is sometimes necessary. In one case, an employee sued the New Jersey Bell Telephone Company, charging that cigarette smoke in the office had seriously irritated her nose, throat, and eyes. In the precedent-setting decision, the company has been ordered to provide special work areas for nonsmokers.

ONE LAST PUFF

Some people return to smoking because they haven't found sufficient substitute rewards. As one persistent smoker told us, "It's one of the few times I feel relaxed. Smoking is one of the few pleasures I'm getting in my life right now — why should I give it up?" In truth, if all the nonsmoker has to look forward to is some extra years of unpleasant life, then it's probably not worth the effort.

But if an attractive, positive addiction can be substituted, the chances of changing that unpleasant life for the better are excellent. That on last puff can mean more than saying goodbye to the bad, it can also be saying hello to some very good, unexpected, and healthful pluses in your life.

7

Malnutrition.

The word makes us think of children with swollen stomachs in Africa or Asia.

But the truth is it is a problem in our culture also — for the rich as well as for the poor.

Many of us, no matter how much we eat, are not getting the right balance of nutrients we need for maximum good health; in many of us deficiencies impair our health, bring on disease, and shorten our lifespans.

We choose foods on the basis of what our culture tells us is good, not on the basis of nutrition. The grocery shelves are stocked with foods that may be good and profitable for the manufacturers but poor for those of us who eat them.

We pay more attention to the quality of the fuel we put in our cars than to the quality of the food we put in our stomachs. We live in a culture that encourages people to eat large amounts of nonnutritious junk foods. Our refrigerators and cupboards are stocked with desserts, snacks, and overprocessed foods. Supermarkets are designed for impulse buying. We spend 40 percent of our food dollars eating out in restaurants, cafeterias, and other places that often encourage us to splurge on rich foods that have little nutritional value. We eat most meals in a hurry and often without even being aware of what we are eating. In one week children may see more than 160 TV ads for sugared cereal, candy, snack foods, and fast-food restaurants, only occasionally seeing an ad for more nutritious foods like fresh vegetables, fruits, milk products.

All these factors contribute to a national diet that recent studies link to at least six of the ten leading causes of death: heart disease, cancer, strokes, diabetes, hardening of the arteries, and cirrhosis of the liver.

Some, but not all researchers also believe our modern diet is often responsible for depression, digestive upsets, fatigue, sexual inadequacies, difficulties in school, tension, anxiety and irritability, and other problems.

More and more evidence accumulates that the excess sugar in our diets is a major factor in the huge increase in diabetes in the United States, now rated with heart disease and cancer as a major killer and crippler. Sugar has been implicated as a factor in many other problems too in both animal and human studies — tooth decay, weight gain, increased blood pressure, bouts of fatigue, hypoglycemia, skin problems including acne, boils and abscesses, spongy gums, and increased tendency to infection.

According to the recent report from the United States Senate Subcommittee on Nutrition and Human Needs, our bad diet represents as great a threat to our health as smoking. We eat too few fruits, vegetables, and whole grains and too much salt, sugar and fat; we drink too much caffeine, and our intake of vitamins and minerals is erratic. The result: hypertension, heart disease, diabetes, fatigue, irritability and depression, and working and living below our potential.

Survey after survey has backed up these statistics, showing our poor diets are both a personal and cultural problem.

A study by the federal Department of Agriculture showed 20 percent of the homes surveyed had poor diets. The White House Conference on Food, Nutrition, and Health reported that 20 million or more Americans are undernourished. Other government studies show the average American consumes over four times as much fat, eight times as much cholesterol, 40 times as much salt and caffeine, and 100 times as much sugar as the body needs. Iron deficiencies are prevalent, especially in women, and fiber consumption is generally low.

One of the greatest concerns is for young children. A study of 642 New York City school children conducted by the city health department showed that 71 percent of the children did not obtain as much as two-thirds of the Recommended Daily Allowances of vitamins and minerals in their diets.

It is difficult to estimate the cost of poor nutrition, but it is probably in the billions. We pay a huge bill for the treatment of the many diet-related diseases, problems that could have been avoided by good nutrition.

But we spend little on nutrition education, promotion and research, either in schools, in government agencies or private institutes.

In fact, a number of nutritionists, including those in the federal Department of Agriculture, say that hundreds of thousands of lives might be saved each year with better nutrition. Good nutrition could possibly add years to our lives, help us ward off disease, give us more energy, and help us enjoy life more. If we just used the knowledge we already have, just applied the most recent facts from research about nutrition, the results could significantly change the practice of medicine, making good eating a prime factor in the prevention and treatment of disease.

Even conservative government nutritionists estimate the following results if our diets were improved: Heart disease and diabetes would be reduced; cancer deaths would decrease; individual IQ and mental alertness would increase. There could be significant benefits for people with dental problems, arthritis, osteoporosis, alcoholism, eyesight deficiencies, allergies, and kidney troubles. Birth defects and pregnancy problems would decline. Millions of the aging could have fewer impairments. Millions of others might be happier, less moody, less irritable, would miss fewer days of work and be more productive.

We did not always have such a poor diet. What we eat and drink daily—and the way we do it—has changed drastically in our culture since the turn of the century. Seventy years ago we ate twice as many of our calories in the form of fruits, vegetables, and whole grains. We ate more complex carbohydrates, less sugar, less salt, and less fat per capita than we do now. In fact, today nearly one-half of our calories come from fats, and about half of the rest come from simple sugars. The result: 30 percent of American men and 40 percent of American women over 40 years of age are obese.

In the last 15 years the change has picked up speed. Many of the foods on our supermarket shelves did not exist in the early 1960's. Our consumption of soft drinks has doubled, edging out milk as the second most consumed beverage. (Coffee is the first.) Processed and convenience foods already account for 50 percent of what we eat, and they are the fastest growing part of the $120 billion food industry. Over 1,300 food additives are used.

Our culture has also influenced the way we eat.

For many of us, commuting takes the time once spent at breakfast and a quick lunch gets us through the day. At dinner we settle down to a big meal, as long as it doesn't take too long to prepare. Armfuls of snacks disappear during the evening in front of the TV.

Much of what we know about nutrition we learn from advertising or the media. The midweek food pages of our newspapers are often filled with recipes reprinted from major food processors and manufacturers. Claims and counterclaims about diets, food additives, research reports, and other nutrition stories jam the news media. A recent study of TV commercials found that 70 percent of the time devoted to food advertising promoted foods high in fat, saturated fat, cholesterol, refined and processed sugar, and salt. Only three percent of the time was devoted to fruits and vegetables—and of that none to vegetables and only seven-tenths of one percent to fresh fruits and juices. Although this was only one study and a limited one, it is a typical finding.

Until recently, formal education and information about nutrition has been lacking. Even most of our doctors learned little about nutrition in their medical schools because it was not considered important. When is the last time a doctor asked you what you eat? The situation is so bad that even the American Medical Association says, "There is inadequate recognition, support, and attention given to this subject in medical schools."

A now-famous Senate report recommends that more be taught to physicians on how to use nutrition and that nutrition education be conducted in high school classrooms and cafeterias across the country and on television. The report also recommends that consumers be given a chance to check nutritional claims in the supermarkets by requiring manufacturers to use more complete labels on their food products.

At present, little research money is going into nutrition to solve areas of controversy and to learn what would truly be best for us to have in our diets. And much of what is learned by the nutrition researchers either never reaches the doctor in practice or is ignored by him because the medical culture at present tends not to give credence to many of the bona fide advances in nutrition treatments. Physicians insist rightly on further research of controversial areas, but they neglect to put into practice the valuable things that have been repeatedly proven. Meanwhile the consumer, often bewildered, tries to gather facts where he can.

One of the most important boosts for good nutrition nationally was the publication of *Dietary Goals for the United States* by the Senate Subcommittee on Nutrition and Human Needs in February and December (revised report) of 1977. While the report caused an uproar among nutritionists, researchers, consumer advocates, doctors, and food companies, most people agree on the overall findings and the general direction of the goals and recommendations. It was the particulars that caused the controversy, pointing up the need for a great deal more research about the quantities of various nutrients and foods. But the main areas in which our national diet is off balance are generally agreed upon, and the United States Dietary Goals gives us one of the best simplified guides to nutritional change that we have.

The goals, very briefly stated, are to:

Avoid overweight
Increase consumption of complex carbohydrates
Reduce consumption of refined and processed sugars
Reduce overall fat consumption
Reduce saturated fat consumption
Reduce cholesterol consumption
Reduce intake of salt

In addition to these goals, the Lifegain program suggests some additional ones that you might want to consider incorporating in your personal goals for change.

Limit or eliminate caffeine consumption (coffee, tea, cola)
Limit alcohol to moderate amounts
Limit or eliminate processed foods, imitation or synthetic foods
Drink four to eight glasses of water a day

A glance at the current United States Diet and the diet we could have if the United States goals were reached, gives us an indication of the cultural pressures that we are all under to eat too much fat and sugar, and too few complex carbohydrates, and gives us some important objectives to reach for as individuals and as a nation (Table 1).

TABLE 1. Components of the U.S. Diet: Where We Are and Where We Could Be

	FAT (PERCENTAGE)	PROTEIN (PERCENTAGE)	CARBOHYDRATE (PERCENTAGE)
Where we are (Current U.S. Diet)	16% saturated 19% monosaturated 7% polysaturated	12%	22% complex carbohydrate 6% "naturally occurring sugar" 18% refined and processed sugar
Total	42%	12%	46%
Where we could be (U.S. Dietary Goals)	10% saturated 10% monosaturated 10% polysaturated	12%	40% complex carbohydrate and "naturally occurring sugar" 10% refined and processed sugar
Total	30%	12%	50%

Note: These percentages are based on calories from food and nonalcoholic beverages. Alcohol adds approximately 210 calories per day to the average diet of drinking-age Americans.

TO GET FROM HERE TO THERE

To reach the proposed goals, the government issued a number of suggestions and recommendations. Simply put they are:

As Individuals

Lose weight if overweight; maintain normal weight if not.

Eat more fruits, vegetables, and whole grains.

Eat less refined and processed sugars and foods high in sugar.

Eat less of foods high in fat, especially saturated fat (substitute polyunsaturated fat).

Eat more poultry and fish, less meat high in animal fat.

Substitute skim or lowfat milk and dairy products for whole milk and highfat dairy products.

Eat less of high cholesterol foods (butterfat, eggs, etc.).

Eat less salt and foods high in salt content.

As a Nation

Provide public money for a public education program to promote the dietary goals for five years—in schools, among school food service workers, in federally funded assistance programs, in Department of Agriculture educational work, in extensive use of television to educate the public.

Require food labeling for all foods, including amounts of cholesterol, salt, calories, percent sugar, percent and type of fats, listing of additives.

Provide public money for studies and pilot projects in food processing and preparation to reduce risk factors.

Increase public funding for human nutrition research.

Give periodic consideration to the implications of nutrition and agricultural policy by a joint committee from Departments of Agriculture and Health, Education, and Welfare.

The Surgeon General's report did not end smoking in the United States. The Senate report cannot end poor nutrition. It takes people to change a culture; and the norms of the supermarket, the restaurants, the eat-on-the-run lifestyle — even our family cultures — cannot change overnight. But it can change. Sweden has begun a ten-year campaign to encourage the public to exercise more and adopt better nutrition patterns. In the first five years sugar consumption has already dropped from 60 to 48 pounds per person per year. (United States consumption is more than 100 pounds.) Fresh vegetable consumption went up from 32 to 45 pounds per year per person.

Here in our country we also can change, as a nation and as individuals. We know what we need to do to meet our daily nutritional needs. But our culture and the national pantry from which we have been selecting our foods have discouraged us from even coming close to meeting these needs.

In this chapter we show you how it can be different; how you can live longer and better, with less impairment and fatigue and more energy and feeling of well-being, by becoming your own nutritionist and making some changes in your diet and in the cultural environments in which you live.

THE LIFEGAIN DIET AND NUTRITION PROGRAM

Step One. Understand Your Own Culture

The first step toward good nutrition is to understand its cultural base. Rather than approaching nutrition as a strictly individual problem, start by really coming to grips with the way in which cultural influences are determining what you eat and figure out what you would like to do about it.

Think about how your culture might be influencing your eating patterns. Do you truly eat the way you would like to so you can feel your best, or do you merely follow those dictates of the culture in which you live?

Check over the following list for culture traps you might be in.

It is a norm in one or more groups that I belong to:

☐ for people to have coffee and a roll, or nothing, instead of a nutritious breakfast in the morning.

☐ for people to eat very little breakfast, more lunch, and a large evening meal.

☐ for people to pay very little attention to the nutritional value of the foods that they eat.

☐ for people to drink a great deal of coffee and other caffeine-based drinks.

☐ for people to eat lots of junk food and prepared convenience foods.

☐ for people to serve sugar-packed cakes, pies, and other rich desserts routinely to guests.

☐ for people to buy unenriched white bread, white flour, white rice, and refined cereals instead of whole grain kinds.

☐ for people at meetings to serve just coffee, sweet rolls, and doughnuts instead of including alternate nutritional snacks.

☐ for many people in the medical profession to neglect the importance of nutrition in helping people to plan better health.

☐ for sweets to be thought of as special treats and therefore more rewarding than most nutritious foods.

☐ for people to eat more than enough calories.

☐ for people to get more starches, fats, sugar, salt, caffeine than they actually need and to be sadly lacking in fiber, vitamins, and minerals.

☐ for people to get infants "hooked" on sugar without realizing the long-range consequences.

☐ for people to feel that anyone who is not overweight can eat anything he wants.

☐ for people to rely on prepackaged, processed foods for most of their food intake.

☐ for people to keep candy, cookies, and sugared sodas in the house for their children.

Now that you think it through, how much does your culture influence your eating patterns and how much is your independent, intelligent choice?

Step Two. Get the Facts and Separate Fact From Fiction

In order to start planning for a change, it is first necessary to get the general facts about nutrition, then the facts about your own nutritional patterns, so that any program you devise is based on sound information.

There is a great deal of conflicting information and controversy concerning nutrition. Sometimes it appears there isn't anything we can eat without someone saying it could be dangerous. Controversy rages over the dangers of sugar, whether foods containing cholesterol are dangerous for the average person, whether you should take vitamin and mineral supplements regularly or not. But most people are agreed that the average American's diet needs great improvement, that many of our ills today could be relieved by improving our diets to correct imbalances and deficiencies, and that, indeed, we could prevent many of these ills from ever happening if we began good nutrition practices early, *before* our problems begin.

In this chapter we try to bring together the most important findings actually shown in research, so you can sort out the facts and make your own decisions.

HOW GOOD AN EXPERT ARE YOU ON NUTRITION?

1. Many affluent Americans suffer from poor nutrition.   True   False
2. The more calories food has, the more nutritious it is.   True   False
3. The body craves what is good for it, so the best way to eat
   is to follow your "natural" likes and dislikes.   True   False
4. Eating sugar is a good way to get quick energy.   True   False
5. One of the best ways to achieve good nutrition is to find
   one basic, highly nutritious food and stick to it.   True   False

1. TRUE. While we tend to think of malnutrition as a problem connected with lack of food, it can also be a result of being overfed or from having the wrong foods.
2. FALSE. Calories are related to the energy that the food produces. Some foods that contain necessary nutrients are actually very low in calories, and some high-caloric foods are "junk."
3. FALSE. A craving for more salt than is good for your body, or for more sugar than is good for your body, can — and often is — easily built up. What seems "natural" often turns out to be cultural. Instead of giving in to the craving, you will be healthier if you re-educate your taste so that your body will like what is good for it.
4. FALSE. Sugar is absorbed quickly and therefore gives you quick energy, but it is not a good source — in fact it can be dangerous to your health, contributing to many problems. Furthermore it has no nutritional value, only calories. Frequent protein snacks or fructose (levulose) sugar can give you steadier, longer-lasting energy.
5. FALSE. There is no one food that can contribute everything you need. The closest to a magic formula for healthy eating is to vary your food as much as possible with intelligent choices from the four basic food groups — meat, milk, vegetable/fruit, bread/cereal — and check for an adequate daily supply of essential nutrients.

SCORE YOURSELF ON YOUR NUTRITION PRACTICES:
Do you eat a well-balanced, nutritious breakfast every day, not
just a doughnut-and-coffee-type breakfast?   Yes   No

Do you eat regular nutritional meals and/or nutritional snacks at regular intervals?	Yes No
Do you avoid processed foods as much as possible?	Yes No
Do you plan your diet in such a way as to include a good balance of the four major food groups?	Yes No
Do you avoid the overuse of sugar, refined starches, caffeine, salt, and fats in your diet?	Yes No
Are you generally aware of the nutritional content of the foods that you eat?	Yes No
Are you aware of the use of vitamin-mineral dietary supplements and have you considered whether you should include them in your diet?	Yes No

If you answered yes to all these questions on nutrition, your body should stand up and publicly thank you. You're doing more for it than most other people are for theirs. If you had any *no* answers and want to improve your looks and how you feel by eating better, you will find hundreds of ideas for better nutrition in the Lifegain nutrition plan in Step Four.

A 48-HOUR NUTRITION TEST

1. For two days keep track of everything you eat, including the number of servings of each. Refer to the chart on page 90 for size of servings (or if you're in a hurry, try to remember everything you ate yesterday, not forgetting snacks, and keep today's count accurately).

   Mark beside each food which of the Four Basic Food Groups it is in.

   Now add up and put on the table below the number of servings you had for each food group, divided by 2, to give you your daily average. Find on the chart the recommended number of daily servings for your category. Finally, note the difference (+1, −2) in number of servings.

NUMBER OF SERVINGS

FOOD GROUP	DAY 1	DAY 2	MY DAILY AVERAGE	RECOMMENDED	DIFFERENCE
Milk/Dairy					
Meat/Protein					
Fruit/Vegetable					
Bread/Cereal					
Others					

Recommended Servings from Four Basic Groups.
The number of servings recommended from each group is based on the amounts of nutrients needed for a 1200 calorie diet.

	RECOMMENDED NUMBER OF SERVINGS				
FOOD GROUP	CHILD	TEEN-AGER	ADULT	PREG-NANT WOMAN	LACTATING WOMAN

Milk
1 cup milk, yogurt, OR
calcium equivalent:
   2 slices (2 oz.) cheddar cheese*
   1 cup pudding
   1¾ cups ice cream
   2 cups cottage cheese*
	3	4	2	4	4

Meat
2 ounces cooked lean meat,
fish, poultry, OR
protein equivalent:
   2 eggs
   2 slices (2oz.) cheddar cheese*
   ½ cup cottage cheese*
   1 cup dried beans, peas
   4 tbsp. peanut butter
	2	2	2	3	2

Fruit–Vegetable ½ cup cooked or juice 1 cup raw Portion commonly served such as medium-size apple or banana	4	4	4	4	4

Grain, whole grain, fortified,
enriched
   1 slice bread
   1 cup ready-to-eat cereal
   ½ cup cooked cereal, pasta, grits
	4	4	4	4	4

*Count cheese as a serving of milk OR meat, not both simultaneously. "Others" comple-ment but do not replace foods from the Four Food Groups. Amounts should be deter-mined by individual caloric needs.

If you find you have a number of servings listed under "other"—and most of us do—look at the foods in this category. Are they foods that are helpful or harmful to your health? The amounts of these should be determined by individual caloric needs. On the chart the recommended servings for adults supply about 1200 calories. You may need more.

In what groups are you lacking? One Lifegain member found she needed one additional serving per day from the fruit/vegetable group and two less servings from the meat/protein group.

2. For the same two days, estimate how many teaspoons of sugar you added to coffee, tea, cereal, or other items. ____ ____

How many sugared drinks did you have each day? ____ ____

How many pieces of candy, pie, cake, or cookies with sugar did you have each day? ____ ____

How much jelly or jam did you eat? ____ ____

Evaluation: You actually don't need any sugar at all. Anything you used was excess, unnecessary, and possibly detrimental to your health, particularly if you are overweight.

3. For the same days, how many cups of coffee, tea or chocolate, or glasses of cola did you have? ____ ____

How many headache pills, cold pills, or other pills containing caffeine did you take? ____ ____

Evaluation: Many doctors find patients (even children) suffering from headache, nervousness, anxiety, and irritability that on investigation turn out to be due to caffeine. If you have more than 4 cups a day, you could be a candidate for this problem.

4. Look over the list of what you ate. How much of it was refined, pre-cooked, or otherwise processed, such as unenriched white bread, white rice, TV dinners, etc., as opposed to being garden fresh, whole, and unprocessed?

Dietary Goals for the United States recommends that as much food as possible be fresh and unprocessed. If less than half of your food is not fresh, you may be missing important nutrients in your diet.

WHAT ARE THE IMPORTANT NUTRIENTS?

While looking at the Basic Four Food Groups will give you some idea about the balance of your diet, it does not get at the problem of foods that are risk factors, and it does not ensure that you are getting the basic nutrients. To get a more comprehensive evaluation of your diet, you will need to have more information about essential nutrients.

While there are about 50 nutrients, including water, that are needed daily for optimum good health, the list can be narrowed down for practical purposes to the ten most important, or "leader nutrients" (Table 2). These are the ones required to be listed on food packages. If you have the proper amount of these leader nutrients in your daily diet, the other 40 or so will most likely occur in sufficient amounts to meet your bodily needs.

WHAT ABOUT VITAMINS AND MINERALS?

An analysis of your vitamin and mineral intake will be an essential part of your total diet analysis. However, there is a great deal of disagreement about

TABLE 2. Nutrients for Health*

NUTRIENT	IMPORTANT SOURCES OF NUTRIENT	SOME MAJOR PHYSIOLOGICAL FUNCTIONS		
		PROVIDE ENERGY	BUILD AND MAINTAIN BODY CELLS	REGULATE BODY PROCESSES
Protein	Meat, Poultry, Fish Dried Beans and Peas Egg Cheese Milk	Supplies 4 Calories per gram.	Constitutes part of the structure of every cell, such as muscle, blood, and bone; supports growth and maintains healthy body cells.	Constitutes part of enzymes, some hormones and body fluids, and antibodies that increase resistance to infection.
Carbohydrate	Cereal Potatoes Dried Beans Corn Bread Sugar	Supplies 4 Calories per gram. Major source of energy for central nervous system.	Supplies energy so protein can be used for growth and maintenance of body cells.	Unrefined products supply fiber — complex carbohydrates in fruits, vegetables, and whole grains — for regular elimination. Assists in fat utilization.
Fat	Shortening, Oil Butter, Margarine Salad Dressing Sausages	Supplies 9 Calories per gram.	Constitutes part of the structure of every cell. Supplies essential fatty acids.	Provides and carries fat-soluble vitamins (A, D, E, and K).
Vitamin A (Retinol)	Liver Carrots Sweet Potatoes Greens Butter, Margarine		Assists formation and maintenance of skin and mucous membranes that line body cavities and tracts, such as nasal passages and intestinal tract, thus increasing resistance to infection.	Functions in visual processes and forms visual purple, thus promoting healthy eye tissues and eye adaptation in dim light.
Vitamin C (Ascorbic Acid)	Broccoli Orange Grapefruit Papaya Mango Strawberries		Forms cementing substances, such as collagen, that hold body cells together, thus strengthening blood vessels, hastening healing of wounds and bones, and increasing resistance to infection.	Aids utilization of iron.
Thiamin (B_1)	Lean Pork Nuts Fortified Cereal Products	Aids in utilization of energy.		Functions as part of a coenzyme to promote the utilization of carbohydrate.

Nutrient	Important Sources	Provide Energy	Some Major Physiological Functions: Build and Maintain Body Cells	Regulate Body Processes
				Promotes normal appetite. Contributes to normal functioning of nervous system.
Riboflavin (B₂)	Liver Milk Yogurt Cottage Cheese	Aids in utilization of energy.		Functions as part of a coenzyme in the production of energy within body cells. Promotes healthy skin, eyes, and clear vision.
Niacin	Liver Meat, Poultry, Fish Peanuts Fortified Cereal Products	Aids in utilization of energy.		Functions as part of a coenzyme in fat synthesis, tissue respiration, and utilization of carbohydrate. Promotes healthy skin, nerves, and digestive tract. Aids digestion and fosters normal appetite.
Calcium	Milk, Yogurt Cheese Sardines and Salmon with Bones Collard, Kale, Mustard, and Turnip Greens		Combines with other minerals within a protein framework to give structure and strength to bones and teeth.	Assists in blood clotting. Functions in normal muscle contraction and relaxation, and normal nerve transmission.
Iron	Enriched Farina Prune Juice Liver Dried Beans and Peas Red Meat	Aids in utilization of energy.	Combines with protein to form hemoglobin, the red substance in blood that carries oxygen to and carbon dioxide from the cells.	Prevents nutritional anemia and its accompanying fatigue. Increases resistance to infection. Functions as part of enzymes involved in tissue respiration.

From "Guide to Good Eating," by the National Dairy Council.

*Nutrients are chemical substances obtained from foods during digestion. They are needed to build and maintain body cells, regulate body processes, and supply energy.

About 50 nutrients, including water, are needed daily for optimum health. If one obtains the proper amount of the 10 "leader" nutrients in the daily diet, the other 40 or so nutrients will likely be consumed in amounts sufficient to meet body needs.

One's diet should include a variety of foods because no *single* food supplies all the 50 nutrients, and because many nutrients work together.

When a nutrient is added or a nutritional claim is made, nutrition labeling regulations require listing the 10 leader nutrients on food packages. These nutrients appear in the chart below with food sources and some major physiological functions.

vitamins and minerals. The government puts out lists of recommended daily allowances (RDA's) which are not acceptable to all parts of the professional community. Some nutritionists say that these should be classified as minimum daily allowances rather than recommended daily allowances.

Because of the great controversy in this area, the authors feel that the most helpful thing for you would be the very basic information on the seven leader vitamins and minerals in the chart below. For more detailed and complete information on all the vitamins and minerals, we refer you to Dr. Jean Mayer's excellent tables in his book, *Diet for Living*, which tell you what each essential vitamin and mineral does for you, what excess or deficiency will mean to you, and the sources for each.

The vitamin story is not in yet. Research in this area is extensive and hopefully much will be clarified in the near future. Your approach now depends on your feeling after getting a good grasp of the pros and cons. Try to read several sources and balance the arguments before making up your mind. Keep in mind that because our food chain is so broken — we often don't know how long "fresh" foods have lingered between the garden and our kitchens; food processing breaks down many nutrients; etc. — we may need more vitamins than we did in the past. On the other hand, more research is needed concerning the effects of extra doses beyond the body's needs.

WHAT ABOUT FIBER?

While relatively little is known about the properties of dietary fiber and its role in nutrition, there is growing evidence that it can be beneficial in helping people avoid diseases of the colon. If you consume a balanced mix of foods with complex carbohydrates making up 48 percent of your diet, the chances are you will get the fiber you need and will not have an excess that could cause mineral deficiency.

ANALYZING YOUR NUTRITIONAL NEEDS

There are a number of different ways to analyze your diet to see if you are getting the proper balance of nutrients your body needs. Trained nutritionists and dieticians can be consulted for a small fee. They usually take a three-day sample of your diet and analyze it for over 50 essentials, then advise you on changes you should make. A list of qualified consultants in your region is available by calling the American Institute of Nutrition (301–530–7050) or by writing the American Dietetic Association (430 N. Michigan Ave., Chicago, Ill. 60611).

Several companies do diet analysis by mail, using a detailed questionnaire on what you eat and how often. A nutrition and activity profile, for example, is done by Pacific Research Systems (2222 Corinth Ave., Los Angeles, Cal. 90064) and Bio Medical Data (P.O. Box 397, West Chicago, Ill. 60185) does diet analysis.

You can also analyze your diet yourself with the help of charts and workbooks available through both the government and private sources. Write to the Government Printing Office, Washington, D.C., for the booklet *Nutrition Labeling* which contains a step-by-step procedure, with sample worksheets and necessary tables of nutrients, which will enable you to make your own analysis of the protein and seven most important vitamins and minerals in nearly 900 foods. A more complete analysis of 441 of these foods is found in *Nutritive Value of Foods*, a Home and Garden Bulletin from the United States Department of Agriculture. This bulletin includes in its analysis fat and fatty acids, carbohydrates, and water content as well as the other leading nutrients. Together they give you all the information and step-by-step procedures that you will need.

Good materials are also available through the National Dairy Council (6300 N. River Road, Rosemont, Ill. 60018) or its affiliate, the Dairy, Food and Nutrition Council, Inc. (172 Halstead St., East Orange, N.J. 07018).

However you choose to obtain an analysis — whether by professional help or by your own blood, sweat and tears — you will then have the basic personal information to use in making a comparison to the good nutritional balance suggested from knowledgeable sources.

Step Three. Find and Build Yourself a Supportive Environment

There are not as many organized support groups for general nutrition as there are for smoking or losing weight, although some are starting in a few communities. Start with your family. Classes in nutrition are sometimes available in colleges, "Y"s, and adult education services. Your doctor may know of a good group in your area, but you may find the best approach is to form your own group, perhaps with other people you know who have read this book or who have heard of the Lifegain program. If you start asking around, it's amazing how many people you'll find who are interested in nutrition, are confused by the controversies, and want to know more.

Bill Johnson, a new warehouse foreman, didn't have time for a formal group, but he found as he talked to people about his new nutrition program that, unknown to him, many friends had been doing some of the same things he had. He suddenly had a new inner fraternity of friends who felt a new closeness because of their interest in nutrition. Simply talking to these other people occasionally, he said, would rekindle his enthusiasm and keep him exploring new facets of nutrition that were of benefit. Bill also found it helpful to check the library for books on nutrition that told him more about scientific investigation in this field.

The more people that you come into contact with who are reaching for the same objectives, the easier it will be for you to adopt your new patterns. The beautiful part is that as the new behavior is supported by other people in your culture it soon becomes the *norm* for that culture. What once was new, different, and even radical now becomes a built-in part of the culture and is self-sustaining.

Consider joining a food co-op that buys nutritious health foods. Many also share ideas and recipes.

Part of building a supportive environment is to see that your pantry and refrigerator are well stocked with nutritious foods and that nonnutritious foods are discarded. Don't give them to your friends — they don't need them any more than you do. Nutritious items that you plan to keep, place in less visible places.

MAKING THE DECISION

You now have analyzed your own eating patterns and found whether there is room for improvement and where.

It is time to make your decision. Check the following boxes as they apply to you:

☐   I have no interest in making a change in my nutrition at this time.

☐   I am seriously committed to making a change and am prepared to improve my nutrition by changing some of the things I eat.

To eat less sugar   ☐

To eat less refined food   ☐

To eat more whole grain natural foods   ☐

To eat more fresh fruits and vegetables   ☐

To reduce my caffeine intake   ☐

To reduce my salt intake   ☐

To change my intake of fat to more healthy levels   ☐

To reduce the animal fat in my diet and substitute some vegetable fats   ☐

To reduce my cholesterol consumption   ☐

To drink more water   ☐

To reduce my alcohol intake   ☐

☐   I am committed to change, but I need more information about my personal nutritional requirements and my current food intake. I plan to further my knowledge so I can evaluate my dietary needs more accurately.

☐   I have demonstrated my commitment to better nutrition by sharing it openly with others and by taking the first steps toward achievement of my goals.

Step Four. Put Your Plan Into Action

You have a number of choices in the kind of plan you follow; the design is up to you. You may want to base a plan on the Four Basic Food Groups, you may want to follow the United States Dietary Goals and the additional dietary goals which expand upon them, or you may want to follow changes recommended by a nutrition counselor. Whatever plan you develop, it needs to be built on sound information — an analysis of your diet with specific foods noted to be added or eliminated — and it needs to incorporate environmental change (your kitchen, your family patterns, your grocery store, and the place you eat outside your home).

TIME OUT FOR NUTRITION!

Whatever your plan, take time out *each day* for good nutrition. You are already spending many hours a day on food shopping, preparing, eating, and cleaning up. An extra few minutes consciously thinking through all of this in relation to good nutrition will pay off in good health. Here are some ways you might spend those additional health-seeking minutes.

As you get into this list of daily suggestions, it will be obvious to you that all these things need not be done, that you are not limited to them, and that they might be done in a different order. We offer them arranged in a daily schedule because some people find it helpful. Feel free to do it your own way.

Day One. Things You Might Do Right Now. Start making some changes in your environment. You could:

Go to the refrigerator and fix yourself a salad.

Throw away junk foods.

Make a list of fresh vegetables and salads to serve tonight and a variety of interesting new nutritious snacks, so you will be surrounded by an environment of nutritious foods to choose from.

If you haven't already done so, call your physician and make arrangements to find out your cholesterol level, to determine if it needs to be lowered.

Talk with the family about trying to have more nutritious snacks and meals; see what kind of changes they feel you all need most.

See if there is a food co-op or other group of people interested in health foods with whom you can share purchases, ideas, and recipes.

Plan a menu for the week. Go through and change all sugar and starch foods to something nutritious.

If you have any medical problems, tell your doctor you are going to change your diet and in what ways. Check to see if you have any chronic conditions that would be affected by the diet or the vitamin supplements or if any medications you are taking might need different dosages on such a diet.

Day Two. Review and Refine Your Plan. If you haven't written down your plan, now is the time to do it. If you have, review it and see how it correlates with these Basic Guides to Good Nutrition. You may want to make some revisions, depending on what dietary changes you have found to be important to you.

10 BASIC GUIDES TO GOOD NUTRITION

1. Eliminate sugar as much as possible. Read labels when you buy so you will not eat any baked, canned, or frozen foods with hidden sugar or any drinks with sugar.
2. Eliminate refined carbohydrates as much as possible, such as unenriched white bread, rice, macaroni, spaghetti, and cakes or cookies. Eat whole grains instead.
3. Eliminate processed foods as much as possible. Eat fresh foods instead of imitation and synthetic junk foods whenever possible.
4. Avoid bacon and processed lunch meats that contain nitrites and nitrates (believed by some to be a factor in causing cancer).
5. Limit fats and oils to moderate amounts. (Don't eliminate them completely; you need adequate amounts for hormones, smooth skin, natural lubrication. But do limit saturated fats.)
6. Limit your intake of coffee, tea, and cola drinks to moderate amounts, especially if you tend to be tense, anxious, or irritable from caffeine or have insomnia. But do drink plenty of liquids.
7. If you use alcohol at all, limit it to moderate amounts.
8. Limit your intake of salt to 5 grams (1 teaspoon) per day. This will keep your sodium down to a safe level and reduce chances of hypertension. This intake, however, only concerns salt you add in cooking or eating. Remember there is a lot of salt already in much of the food you buy — not only on pretzels, potato chips, etc., but in canned and processed foods. If sodium is a particular concern of yours, you will need to take all these into account also.
9. Eat as much variety as you can from the four food groups: whole grains such as seed, brown, and wild rice, whole wheat, wheat germ, and other whole grain products; all kinds of fruits, salads, vegetables, potatoes, berries, melons (fresh when possible instead of canned or frozen); fish, shellfish, poultry and eggs, dried beans and peas, meats (broil, bake, or roast, instead of frying); all kinds of cheese and yogurt (except kinds that have sugar added).
10. Unless you feel sure you are eating a well-balanced diet of fresh unprocessed foods, consult with your doctor or nutritionist about proper balance and amounts of vitamins and minerals, particularly those listed as most frequently missing in today's United States diet.

Day Three. Start Buying for the Best Nutrition. Make a shopping list for the next few days. Then go back over it, keeping in mind your plan and the Lifegain diet rules. Make the necessary changes to keep it in tune with them. Here are some pointers:

- What you buy goes into your stomach.
- Don't have candy, cookies, and other empty calories in the house.
- Get as wide a variety of foods as possible, since different foods contain different nutrients.
- Buy fresh food when possible instead of canned or frozen (though frozen food can be better than old, poorly cared for "fresh" produce that has lain around too long).
- As you start to switch your eating patterns around, load your house with every appetizing snack you can think of so you won't get bored and restless looking for the usual junk food.
- Visit a health food store. See if there is anything there that appeals to you: papaya juice, sunflower seeds, kelp. Buy according to an intelligent plan. Don't buy everything in sight—even "health" stores sometimes overadvertise and overcharge.

And when you go to the store, allow more time for shopping (in fact, do this for the next few weeks) so that you can really study the produce and health food sections, read the labels, and choose foods selectively and wisely. (On labels, ingredients are listed in order of the relative quantity.)

Day Four. Making Some Healthy Substitutes. The next time you go shopping keep these possibilities in mind:

If You Have Been Using	Use Instead
Meat, with fat	Meat, lean
Fried meat or meat pot pie	Broiled meat
Lunch meats with nitrites	Leftover meats of your own
Oil-packed food	Water-packed food
Canned fruit in syrup	Fresh fruit, or packed in juice only
White bread	High protein, whole wheat, rye, or gluten bread
White rice	Brown rice or bean sprouts
Pearled barley	Whole grain barley
Refined wheat flour	Soya flour (use ½ amount wheat flour called for in recipe) or whole wheat, whole grain rye, whole grain buckwheat, cornmeal
Pudding	Fruit cocktail or no-sugar gelatin
Sherbet	Fruit slush or fresh fruit ice
Ice cream	Frozen yogurt without sugar
Junk snacks	Nuts, raisin, fruits
Junk cereal	Whole grain or home-cooked cereals
Coffee	Decaffeinated coffee or weak tea
Sucrose sugar	Fructose sugar
Canned or precooked foods	Fresh foods
Hydrogenated peanut butter	Pure natural peanut butter
Salt	½ salt/½ potassium (now available in grocery stores)

Day Five. Review Your Cooking and Food Preparation Behavior
- Fix a good breakfast including fruit or fruit juice, whole grains or eggs.
- Keep lots of fresh fruits and vegetables cleaned, attractively prepared, and easy to grab. Have other healthy snack food handy to eat between meals: cheese, nuts, leftover poultry or meats.
- Keep the vitamin and mineral supplement right on the kitchen counter at all times so it's easy to take your daily supply in the morning at breakfast.
- Don't overcook things. Eat things garden fresh when possible.
- Cook with as little water as possible. Sometimes use alternate methods: braise, cook in a Chinese wok, bake potatoes, steam vegetables. Try to use leftover cooking water when you can for soups or stews. Use leftover vegetables like asparagus, beans, beets, peas in salads the next day instead of cooking them again and causing more nutrient loss.

Day Six. Review What's Happening To You. It's not too soon to draw back from details for a few minutes and take a larger view of what's going on. Here are some things to consider:

√ *Make sure you are eating plenty.* Sometimes when people eliminate sugars and starches there doesn't seem to be anything left in the house to eat, and they end up feeling hungry and restless, or even weak. Eat! Just don't eat junk. But switch to fruits, vegetables, salads, cheeses, nuts, and meats.

Especially continue to eat a good breakfast.

And go ahead and nibble, as long as you are not getting more calories than you should. Research with animals shows that animals fed many times a day gain less weight than those fed the same total amount of food in only three meals. Many people find it very helpful during this diet changeover period to eat a protein snack of cheese, meat, or nuts every three hours for long lasting energy. Just make sure your snacks are not weight-producing sweets and starches.

√ *If you have started vitamin and mineral supplements.* Remember that vitamins and minerals and diet do not work alone, but work as a team with one another. So be sure to keep up the good diet if you take supplements. By beginning the new diet and supplements separately you can tell how each is affecting you. No one thing works for everybody. The true test for anything is whether it works for you. If at any time you have a bad reaction to a diet or to a vitamin, simply stop using it. But chances are you're feeling super already.

Day Seven. Think About How Much Salt You Use. Most people use 20 to 30 times more salt than they need. High salt intake can cause the body to retain liquid, sometimes causing the heart to work harder, and it may be a factor in high blood pressure.

If you have high blood pressure, kidney disease, premenstrual tension, or periodically have swollen boggy ankles, feet, hands, or other parts, you should talk to your doctor about ways to cut down your salt intake.

If you want to cut down: don't eat foods with high salt content such as canned soups, pickled items, or salty snack foods; don't add salt when you cook; use spices and herbs as alternate seasonings.

You can now buy prepared mixes that are half salt and half potassium. This helps you cut down your salt. If you oversalt, the taste tells you.

If you cut salt down gradually you probably won't miss it. It is amazing how much you can cut down and how little you even notice the decrease when it is done this way.

You can check the family salt use by dating the new container, then, after it is used up, dividing the total ounces by each day. Using the suggested goal of one teaspoon per day per person, you can see if your family average is way off. Of course, this does not take into account salted pretzels, peanuts, etc. Hopefully, by now you will have found unsalted substitutes for these nibblers.

Day Eight. Fix Something Special. It's time to please yourself and prove to yourself that nutritious eating can still be exciting eating.

Experiment with foreign or gourmet recipes to wake up your nutrition interest and get out of an eating rut.

Have a luscious melon for dessert or frozen yogurt with fruit on top.

Please yourself with exotic appetizers and fruit punch to liven up what might have been a routine cocktail hour before dinner.

Get some bean or alfalfa seeds, put them in a glass bottle, rinse them every day with fresh water, and watch them sprout. They are wonderfully nutritious and good to add to salads.

Try baking something yourself using whole grain flours and artificial sweeteners instead of sucrose.

Check the vitamin-mineral chart for good foods that are rich in special nutrients. Perhaps you can work them into a special dish.

Day Nine. Check Your Progress. You should be feeling a new sense of energy already. Most people do. But if you have any side effects (they can occur with even the best of diets), check with your doctor.

Continue the Basic Steps of the Lifegain Diet. Continue shopping and cooking to obtain the most nutrients. Continue treating yourself by having lots of good foods and nutritious snacks and drinks in the house.

WHEN YOU HAVE YOUR NEXT CHECKUP

Have your doctor compare your cholesterol, triglyceride, glucose, uric acid, and blood pressure values with your previous readings so you can judge any effect your diet or other factors are having. And think about the symptoms you complained of at your last checkup and whether they have improved or even disappeared.

You should be pleasantly surprised.

Discuss your diet with your doctor and see if he has any further suggestions for ways you could improve it even more.

Special Plans for Special Problems

IF YOU HAVE DIGESTIVE PROBLEMS

If you frequently get indigestion, heartburn, belching, bloating, gas, abdominal pain, cramps, constipation, or diarrhea, you should see your doctor to determine the cause. You could have a serious disease requiring treatment, or you may be under tension that is affecting you. But it may be as simple as your diet.

- Analyze what in your diet seems to bring on the attacks: fat, sugar, caffeine, milk? When you suspect a food or drink, eliminate it from your diet for a week or two, and see if there is a difference.
- Try eliminating all sweets and starches and substituting a high fiber diet, with whole grain bread, whole grain cereal, fruit, and vegetables.
- Try eliminating alcohol from your diet.

IF YOU HAVE HIGH CHOLESTEROL LEVELS

High levels of cholesterol in the blood have definitely been associated with fatty deposits in the arteries and with the occurrence of heart attacks and strokes. But you need some cholesterol for production of hormones and other vital substances and to keep your skin, your menstrual cycles, your sex life, and other body functions working properly.

The general belief among most physicians at this time is that *everyone* does not need to reduce cholesterol. If your level is normal, you can continue to eat some high cholesterol foods like eggs and shrimp because they have an abundance of good nutrients. But if your blood level of cholesterol is high, you will want to work with your physician on changing your diet to get the level down. You may find it decreases tremendously when you go on the Lifegain nutrition program and begin an exercise program.

New data show that there are actually three forms of cholesterol being transported about your body: two bad kinds and one good kind. Whether they are good or bad depends on the way the cholesterol fat is chemically hooked up with a protein to be carried through the bloodstream.

The good cholesterol form is high density lipoprotein (HDL). Researchers find the more HDL you have, the *less* are your chances of having heart disease or a stroke. The HDL form of cholesterol actually seems to *prevent* heart attacks and stroke.

The bad cholesterol forms are called low density lipoprotein (LDL) and very low density lipoprotein (VLDL). They *increase* the risk of coronary heart disease.

What all this means is that now when you have your cholesterol level tested, your doctor should request the more sophisticated test that gives the levels of good kinds and bad kinds.

Many people may be following a strict diet or taking drugs when they do not need to. They should learn what *kinds* of excess cholesterol they have.

How to raise your HDL and lower your LDL? So far research shows some people are able to do it by taking lecithin, eating fish, exercising, keeping their proper weight, not smoking, and not drinking heavily.

Other ways to reduce cholesterol: Eliminate sugar and refined starches from your diet; eat lots of fruits and vegetables for their natural pectin, recently shown in England to be very effective in lowering cholesterol levels; eat whole fiber foods; take adequate amounts of vitamins A, B, and C; and decrease the stress in your life.

IF YOU ARE TAKING BIRTH CONTROL PILLS

If you take birth control pills that contain estrogen or you take estrogen for menopause or other reasons, you may need extra supplements of vitamins B_6 and B_{12}, niacin, folic acid, and vitamin C. Some doctors also recommend vitamins A and E.

Taking the supplements not only can help to restore the normal balance of vitamins and minerals in the body, but it often alleviates symptoms of nausea, dizziness, depression, and swelling that estrogen users frequently have.

IF YOU ARE PREGNANT

Women who are pregnant need many extra nutrients, especially folic acid and iron. Go to a doctor for vitamins and mineral supplements and diet advice the minute you suspect you are pregnant. It can be vital for both you and your baby.

IF YOU THINK YOU ARE ALLERGIC

If a food seems to bring on attacks of indigestion, heartburn, belching, bloating, gas, abdominal pain, cramps, constipation, diarrhea, hives, or other reactions, you may be allergic to it. Eliminate it from your diet for a week or two and see if your symptoms disappear. Then eat it again and see if the symptoms reappear.

If you have established a food allergy, watch out for related foods also.

Step Five. Keep Track and Tune In

While it isn't always easy, it's very important to keep track of results as you change your eating habits. Check back regularly and ask yourself how well you have kept up with your objectives. After a month look over the tests on pages 88–91 and see your improvement. Refer back frequently to the 10 Basic Guides to Good Nutrition or post the list in your kitchen to see how well you're doing.

Mentally go through your meals and snacks for the previous few days and score yourself on how well you handled your eating. If the entire family is trying to improve eating patterns, you can have a family meeting each week for several weeks and discuss everyone's progress. Also give reports on any negative nutrition norms you each may have avoided or changed at work, school, with organizations, or friends.

The checking that is most satisfying is to tune into yourself. Go over the symptoms that were bothering you when you started on this program and see if after two weeks any have improved. Check again in 30 days for further improvement. If you break your diet, notice if any of your symptoms come back or get worse. Also compare results on specific tests the next time you go to your doctor. See if your cholesterol levels have dropped, or high blood pressure or other problem areas have improved.

Step Six. Reward Yourself and Have Fun

Don't get so enthusiastic about your new eating regimen that you forget how to enjoy eating. Eating is fun, and you can keep it that way with healthy, great dishes so that staying with the new eating pattern will be rewarding for you. Reward yourself, and your friends and family, with special treats and gourmet dishes. You can still bake, just use fructose or artificial sweetener and whole wheat flour instead of white flour. At least once a month make or ask for something special that you haven't enjoyed before on this diet.

And most people are rewarded by feeling so much better and by getting rid of symptoms that have bothered them for years that they don't ever want to go back to their old habits.

An extra bonus: Eating the freshest and least-processed foods is often cheaper than eating the processed and convenience foods. Use the money you save to do other things you'd like. So you can eat like a gourmet and save money on your food budget, then use the money you save to double your enjoyment with a second reward.

Step Seven. Reach Out To Others

FAMILY BUSINESS

You may want to start your reaching-out program with your family. Talk over the things you have learned in this chapter with your family. As a family project you might check just how much sugar your family is consuming.

For two days check the foods that each person eats to see how much sugar is really being consumed. Keep track of candy, chewing gum, soft drinks, tea, coffee, or chocolate with sugar, cakes, pies, cookies, donuts, sugared cereal, jams and jellies. Don't forget to ask what they ate at school, at friend's houses, and for snacks. Also read the labels on canned or frozen foods you've eaten where there is an amazing amount of sugar added in processing.

One study of teenagers in Iowa showed that the average sugar intake for girls was 55 teaspoons per day, and for boys was 78 teaspoons per day. Some consumed more than 100 teaspoons per day, amounting to 400 pounds per year.

Once you realize how much sugar your family is consuming, you may wish to make a real effort to help your family members change their eating patterns.

You may also want to check on your family's caffeine consumption. The United States Senate report expressed concern over the amount of caffeine ingested by children, especially in cola drinks, which pediatricians report can cause irritability, headaches, and nervousness.

Other things you can do with your family:

See that everyone has a good breakfast before going to work or school. They need energy to get them through the morning. Studies done of school children in Iowa showed a definite increase in work capacity and better attitude toward schoolwork when they had an adequate breakfast.

Don't keep candy, cookies, cakes, pies, and sugared drinks in the house; they won't be missed that much. Red Buttons and his wife Alicia serve unprocessed millet or oatmeal with fresh-squeezed orange juice for breakfast, and snacks may be fruits, nuts, or sunflower seeds, and the kids love it, they say.

Don't worry if your children eat things at weird times, as long as they eat good things. And don't worry if young children drink a lot of water. They need extra fluids. Let them eat between meals if they wish, but make the snacks nutritious. Children feel hungry more often than adults, but cannot eat as much at one sitting.

Set up a self-service snack center — one or two shelves in the refrigerator where everyone knows to reach and on the counter next to the refrigerator, both filled with nutritious and grabable foods. To top it off, you might want to put a small bulletin board with a list or chart of diet guidelines and with space where people can stick suggestions for future snacks, things that need buying, or clippings of super-looking new foods or recipes to try.

Allowable treats: milk, fruit juices, cottage cheese, yogurt, cheeses of all kinds, leftover meats, melon slices or dishes of melon balls, carrot and celery sticks, cauliflower buds, radishes, cabbage leaves, sliced green peppers, cherry tomatoes, tangerines, apples, oranges, grapefruit, bananas, dried apricots, dates, figs, prunes, little boxes of raisins, whole wheat crackers, or whole grain bread. In the freezer you might have individual containers of frozen yogurt. Extra nice: a stack of paper plates, napkins and glasses on the counter too. The trick is to have everything prepared and attractively grabable.

Also reward members of your family as they reach a particular goal in regard to nutrition, such as cutting out salty, fatty snacks for a week or giving up sugar-coated cereals. And set up rewards for family members who succeed in influencing someone else. One family took the norm indicator and counted their negative nutrition norms. At the end of a month they did it again. For every negative norm changed they put a dollar in the pot and spent it on a family outing.

FRIENDS, GUESTS, AND FELLOW WORKERS

You will also want to reach out to others beyond your family.

Keep to your good nutrition program when you have guests, not serving heavy, gooey, or sweet desserts just because you think they expect it. Serve attractively prepared yogurt or fruit or melon and see how well these desserts are received.

Be the first one in your block to have a frozen yogurt maker—now available in small appliance sections—and treat the neighborhood to cones some hot summer evening.

Have you tried getting some of the organizations to which you belong to serve something besides coffee and cake at their meetings? (One group changed the name from "coffee break" to "energy break" and served cheeses, cold meats, fruits, and juices.) Or you could choose lunch and dinner menus for meetings that are more nutritious than the usual standard meeting fare.

Have you tried to reach out and get your office to serve something else for coffee break instead of coffee and rolls?

What about your office cafeteria? Can you talk to the manager about serving more fresh fruits and vegetables, using less salt, putting attractive healthful foods up front, and putting the sugar-laden desserts in back? Some people have formed committees in their companies to work with the cafeteria people, helping them to meet nutritional needs better.

If you know someone who is sick or about to go into the hospital for surgery, have you suggested to them that they talk to their physician about taking supplementary vitamins and minerals.

If you are a physician you could seek some additional training in the latest nutrition research and see that your patients are practicing good nutrition. And if you have seen the nutritional approaches work with your patients, you might suggest a program or class on nutrition in the hospital or medical school you are affiliated with.

INTO THE SCHOOLHOUSE

You may want to check on what your school's lunch program is like also. The United States Department of Agriculture sampled school lunches in 300 schools and found 15 percent of the lunches were lacking in calcium, two-thirds were low in iron, one-third were low for vitamin A, more than a third were high for fat. That's what was put on the trays. The children's intake was even worse when you figured the vegetables, fruit, and other foods that went into the garbage pail. And some students skip a regular lunch to have a candy bar, a soft drink, or a milk shake. Perhaps, through your Parent—Teachers Association, you can have some influence on the lunches in your school. You might give a copy of this book to your child's teacher for possible incorporation into the science or health program, or if you are a teacher, try discussing the Lifegain approach with your class.

You could try to get your school to have fruit, nuts, diet sodas, and fruit juices in the snack machines instead of just sugared colas and candy. In one school, lunches were planned to please the kids and be nutritious, including beef and cheese tacos; salads; cheese pizzas with wheat germ added; meat and bean burritos; fried chicken; cheeseburgers with wheat germ in the buns; sandwiches with one slice of whole wheat and one slice of white bread.

In a school in Milwaukee the student council plans the meals, then by offering only one meal gets twice the usual consumption by students, and at about half the usual price. Another school uses fast food packaging but adds vitamins, uses only unrefined flour, eliminates additives. Prices are lower for the package deals and the students end up with salads too. Others offer a mix-it-yourself salad bar.

Have you explored the possibility of your P.T.A. or other group having a speaker and discussion on nutrition?

All of these suggestions are meant to stimulate your thinking so you can generate your own ideas on how to reach out. Most important of all, none of these will work all by themselves if they are merely laid on top of a culture that supports poor nutrition. The answer, it appears from our experience, lies in working with each group you belong to — your family, work place, community, etc. — systematically involving people in examining their own cultural biases. People can and will substitute good nutritional norms when they have a chance to consider the alternatives.

Good nutritional norms can be a lot more acceptable in our society than most of us had up until now thought possible.

8

How To Stay Slim for Life

Imagine a documentary film. The plot is simple, the cast large: a culture in which as many as 80 percent of the people are overeating, encouraging fatigue, illness, even death.

The film shows that from childhood people are encouraged to eat more than they need. Doting grandparents admire pudgy babies and pronounce them healthy. Teenage weight is excused as baby fat. Many adults regularly go on special diets to slim down to fit into fashionable clothes, but heavy eating and drinking usually take over again. By middle age, most people become less active, keep the same eating patterns, and start putting on pounds they will never permanently lose.

Food, the film shows, often seems to be involved with other things besides energy and nutrition. It's a norm in the culture for people to eat to relieve anxiety or for recreation, to go out to dinner, to invite friends over for dessert, to take a coffee break during the day. When people sit down to watch TV they automatically reach for snacks. They use food for rewards, offering lollipops to children who behave and a second helping of homemade apple pie to someone who's finally lost weight. They celebrate special occasions with cakes or big meals.

Right in the middle of the film is a dramatic sequence — time-lapse photography, using a series of slides taken over time to show the eating practices the culture encourages, the weight it adds year-by-year, and the health problems it aggravates. The flashing slides show the weight gain over the years is a slow process. Some call it the "creeping" sickness — one meal, one pie, one cake, one coffee break, one TV snack, one Thanksgiving at a time over a period of years. All the still pictures of second helpings, party drinks, morning Danish, evening nibbles, and holiday desserts flash like an animated cartoon on the screen. And as the foods disappear, the fat and all that goes with it appears.

The culture is our own. More of us than we like to realize are starring in the film. Our culture has cast us in the uncomfortable role of overeaters. It has us on a slow motion overeating binge that gradually adds pounds for each of us individually while at the same time it is increasing our *average* weight. The average American is not only overweight, he and she are *more* overweight than they were 10 years ago. We've been slowly losing the war on fat. And the average American is now 20 to 30 pounds overweight.

Thanks to the slow motion eating binge our culture encourages, overweight afflicts more of us than probably any other health problem. We range from being a few pounds over the recommended weight for our height and body type to being life-threateningly obese. And despite the popularity of weight loss diets, the problem is growing.

Most of us at one time or another have tried to lose weight. We often have great success. But keeping it off is another story. Some people can lose 1,000 pounds and still be overweight, because they lose it over and over but keep gaining it back again.

It's much too easy in our culture to overeat and to eat the wrong things.

We gain weight when we eat more than our bodies require to supply our own special energy needs. Height, physical condition, age, body type, and the amount of exercise we get all determine how much food energy, measured in calories, we need. The body is geared either to make use of what we eat or store it as fat. It never forgets a nibble. Eat two or three slices of dry toast more than you need every day and you can add 10 pounds in a year.

But dry toast is the least of the temptations the culture offers. With donuts, pastries, butter and rolls for breakfast and coffee breaks, most of us could eat all the calories we need before lunch.

For millions of years humans had the opposite problem, not enough food. In some cultures here and abroad, it is still a problem. But most of us have more than enough. Our culture has not caught up. We have held onto the norms that helped in a time when there were frequent food shortages and people spent large amounts of energy in walking, working, and other forms of exercise. But they no longer work for us.

Excessive weight increases the likelihood that we will have high blood pressure, heart disease, diabetes, strokes, gallbladder problems, hypertension, and cancer. The extra pounds can damage weight-bearing bones and joints, aggravating gout or arthritis. Menstrual disorder and uterine cancer are more frequent among obese women. A person 30 percent overweight is four times more likely to die before a person of the same age and the proper weight.

Even those of us only a few pounds overweight suffer from these problems. The immediate effect is to make one part of our life or another less enjoyable and productive. We may feel uncomfortable in a bathing suit. Or we may drag at the end of the day, after lugging around our extra suit of flab. It's like carrying a suitcase with you all day long seven days a week, 52 weeks a year. And the same culture which encourages us to overeat also blames us for it. We may believe we're unattractive, play the straight man or woman for overweight jokes at parties, lose a promotion. Most people begin to put on weight more rapidly in their middle years. It heightens the sense of feeling old before our time. And even if we do not experience any problems right now because of our tendency to overeat and underexercise, it does not mean we will not. Most of us don't put on 20 or 30 pounds in one year. It creeps on at the rate of a half-pound to a pound a month.

The culture as a whole makes it easy to gain weight.

We are bombarded with stimuli encouraging us to eat. Advertisements push food by equating it with everything from good sex to good health. Actors are carefully chosen who do not have a weight problem, no matter how much highfat food they eat in 30 seconds. Fast food stores line the highways. Prepared high caloric foods crown supermarket shelves and fill our refrigerators. Big meals weigh down our tables.

Our butchers leave fat on our steaks. We overload our table when we have guests to show our affluence and our generosity. Our supermarket checkout aisles are filled with junk food while nutritional foods are given much less prominent displays.

Some of us stuff ourselves as if we were still back on the farm; but we're no longer working and burning calories as we were back on the farm.

From the first day of birth some of us give our babies sugar water. We consider fat babies cute babies. We urge the baby to finish the bottle and children to clean their plates, whether they are full or not. We add sugar to their food. We give them cookies for being good, cakes on their birthday, and even doctors give out lollipops after the child gets a shot. We have ice cream stores in every neighborhood and bakeries that only offer confections of white flour and sugar, never of whole grain flour. Bread and catsup and sometimes even salt has sugar added to it. We give candy as gifts to hostesses, to mothers on Mother's Day, and on other holidays. Who would think on Valentine's Day we would express love by giving someone extra calories and harmful sugar?

It all contributes to a national diet high in sugar, fat, and cholesterol. Sugar is the most common food additive. So-called "natural" cereals contain more sugar ounce for ounce than soft drinks. Our average sugar consumption is 128 pounds per year. We do not require any. Our average "fat" bill is 10 to 30 percent higher than it needs to be. We pay the price in heart disease, which is eight times more common than it should be.

Those are the ways in which the culture as a whole influences us. The influence of smaller groups, from our families to those with whom we may share an ethnic heritage, also greatly influence our eating patterns.

Research shows that overweight is associated with education, sex, race, and wealth. Men with high incomes tend to be 20 percent fatter than those who earn less. Men with a college education are 10 percent heavier than high school graduates. Women follow almost the reverse pattern. Wealthy women are 20 percent thinner than their husbands and 20 percent thinner than women who never went to high school.

Black American men are thinner than white American men, but black women are heavier. Americans of British descent tend to be thinner than those from an Eastern European background.

What we do about our weight problems is also culturally determined.

The word "diet" has been redefined by our culture. It no longer means "our usual food and drink" as the dictionary defines the word. It has come to mean something you do when you want to lose weight.

We go on weight-loss diets—and off them—frequently. We live in a culture that has made weight loss part of the whole weight-gain cycle.

But despite the popularity of "going on a diet," chances are that weight lost will be regained, even for those who do it under a doctor's supervision. Of all the people who ask a doctor to help them lose weight, relatively few actually keep their weight loss. Once exposed to the norms of the overeating culture, they gain their weight back again in one or two years. Most people who try to lose weight have done it dozens of times, losing the same pounds over and over again.

From the way it tells us to take it off to the way it encourages us to put it on, the culture—from our families to the food industry—supports the fattening of America.

We eat donuts for breakfast, drink milkshakes and colas for lunch, and consider dessert the most exciting part of dinner. We keep eating after we are full so that we do not insult our hostess or our mother. We fill our cupboard with candy and cookies for snacks.

Hank Pacelli knows what it's like to gain and lose and gain again.

"I lost 30 pounds under a doctor's care, but within a year and a half, I was back up."

"It was always just 'You do it'," Hank recalls.

Then he tried one of the popular weight control programs, but he felt something was missing—real concern and support.

"A professional measures you to see how you are doing. It takes maybe 10 seconds. The group I was in had 50 people in it," Hank recalls.

Now Hank is in a Lifegain weight-loss program. He says that he now realizes that his family was not supporting his efforts to lose weight.

That's changed. He and his wife now plan meals together and take brisk half-hour walks in the evening. A son in college calls every week to check on his progress and offer support.

"I'm taking a relaxed long-range approach," he says.

"My goal is to lose about 25 pounds in six months. In two months I'm down 10 pounds. I think it's going to accomplish not only weight loss but change the way I eat."

Everywhere we go we meet negative norms that make it hard for us, even when we have sincerely decided we want to stay slim for life.

The norms trap us into expecting a constant cycle of weight loss and weight gain. But if we want to end the slow motion fattening permanently, we need to study our own culture to see how it affects us, then change it around, so we can have a stay-slim diet for life.

Step One. Understand Your Own Culture

The first step in an effective, long-range weight control program is to understand its cultural basis. How many negative norms are in your culture? How heavily do they influence you? What would be the effect if all these norms were positive?

Read through the following norm indicator to see what cultural norms might be helping to keep you overweight. It lists some of the most prevalent negative norms of weight control. These norms may or may not exist in the groups with which you are associated. Check off those you see as norms — expected, accepted, and supported behavior — for the people in your groups.

It is a norm in one or more groups that I belong to:

☐ For people to see children who are slightly overweight as healthier and better cared for than children who aren't.

☐ For most people to be a few pounds overweight.

☐ For people to see desserts such as cake, pie, pudding, and ice cream as a usual part of the lunch or dinner menu.

☐ For sweets to be thought of as special treats and therefore more "rewarding" than most nutritious foods.

☐ For parents to encourage children not to leave food on their plates, even if it is more than they want or need.

☐ For people to associate overindulging in food with relaxation, pleasure, and good social relationships.

☐ For hosts and hostesses to encourage guests to eat more food than would be desirable for them.

☐ For people to view the offer of large food portions as a sign of generosity.

☐ For people to look at being slightly overweight as "natural," particularly among older people.

☐ For people to eat more food than they want or need.

☐ For people to lose weight through dieting but gain it right back again.

☐ For people to find pie eating, watermelon eating, and other eating contests to be amusing parts of our culture.

☐ For people to think or say everybody loves a fat person.

☐ For people to think it's natural to be overweight if you belong to certain ethnic groups.

☐ For people to eat when they're lonely or their feelings are hurt.

☐ For people to feed children more than they need for growth and health because it shows that you love them.

Ask yourself if these, or any other factors, are affecting your attitude toward food. By recognizing and understanding them, you can learn to deal with them and not let them undermine your efforts.

Keep practicing that flash of recognition as the culture trap clicks. "You're on a diet? Oh, but you can break it this once." *Click.* "Come on, have another piece of cake. I worked for hours this afternoon making it just for you." *Click.* (Maybe two clicks — she's trying to lay guilt on you too.)

Step Two. Get the Facts and Separate Fact From Fiction

HOW MUCH DO YOU REALLY KNOW ABOUT WEIGHT AND WEIGHT CONTROL?

Count your facts before you count your calories.

There are many misconceptions about food and dieting, and those misconceptions can often mean the difference between success and failure in losing weight.

Assess your knowledge about weight and weight control with the following true-false quiz.

Questions:

1. It's natural to get fatter as you get older.   True   False
2. It makes no difference whether a person eats slowly or quickly.   True   False
3. Toasting reduces the calories in bread.   True   False
4. Alcohol furnishes calories to the body.   True   False
5. People who overeat are simply hungrier than those who eat less.   True   False
6. Although exercise is a good thing, it cannot contribute much toward helping us reduce our weight and maintain our proper weight level.   True   False
7. The best way to lose weight is by cutting back all your food intake drastically.   True   False
8. The most important factor in weight control for most people is not heredity or glands but the individual's handling of food.   True   False
9. If you don't succeed in reaching the weight indicated for you on the standard weight chart, you've failed.   True   False
10. If you're embarking on a program of extensive weight reduction, the first thing to do is skip at least one of the three meals you ordinarily eat each day.   True   False
11. Being overweight can be a contributing factor to such problems as heart disease, diabetes, and hypertension.   True   False
12. Exercise will only make me eat more.   True   False
13. A person who eats too much is more likely to be getting the vitamins and minerals he needs than someone who eats less.   True   False
14. If you can lose those extra pounds just once, you can go back to eating the way you do now because you aren't gaining weight now.   True   False
15. Most people gain weight when they stop smoking, so it is better to go on smoking rather than get fat.   True   False

Answers:

1. FALSE. Many people do grow fatter as they get older, but it is not natural or necessary. As a person grows older, metabolism and physical

activity often decrease. Fat begins to accumulate as the person takes in, day after day, more food than his body uses. The answer: eat less and exercise more.

2. FALSE. Most overweight people eat quickly. They consume large amounts of food without even realizing it. One should always eat slowly and chew food well. This gives the sugar regulatory mechanisms of the body a chance to act on our appetite-regulating centers to allow us to be satisfied.

3. FALSE. Burning the bread destroys some nutritive value but does not burn away the calories.

4. TRUE. A whiskey or a pint of beer is the caloric equivalent of a slice of bread and butter or an average portion of potatoes.

5. Only sometimes. Actually many people who overeat do a lot of eating after their hunger is already satisfied.

6. FALSE. It *can* contribute a good deal, but it takes a while. To work off one pound of fat takes seven and one-half hours of bicycling, but the effects are cumulative. An hour a day bike ride means a pound a week. The best combination is exercise *plus* lower calorie intake.

7. FALSE. It's not how much you eat, it's *what* you eat. In addition, a drastic reduction in intake is rarely effective in long-range weight control, as it cannot be maintained. And it is often unhealthy, since you don't get proper nutrients.

8. TRUE. While there are isolated cases of persons whose weight control is seriously affected by heredity or disease, for most people the control of their weight is in their own hands.

9. FALSE. First, the ideal weight for you may be somewhat higher or lower than that on the chart. Second, if you are 40 pounds overweight and manage to get down to 20 pounds overweight, you are that much better off. Fifty percent success may not be as good as 100 percent, but it's certainly better than nothing.

10. FALSE. Usually skipping meals is not a good idea. It is better to cut down on high caloric, high carbohydrate foods. Actually, the first thing you should do is consult your physician.

11. TRUE. Overweight can contribute to the onset of these and other illnesses or aggravate and magnify their effects.

12. FALSE. Studies have shown that, if anything, regular exercise tends to reduce excess food intake. And strangely, one study shows a little exercise tends to make you eat more, but more exercise tends to make you eat less.

13. FALSE. Many of the foods we eat today are empty calories having virtually no nutritional value at all. The quantity of food eaten has no necessary relation to the nutritional quality.

14. FALSE. What is a maintenance diet for your present weight will be a weight gaining diet when you get to a lower weight. Once you get to your desired weight the best way to stay there is to eat the maintenance diet for that weight.

15. FALSE. The typical weight gain of a withdrawing smoker totals about seven pounds, an amount not really difficult to lose. It has been calculated that the bad physical effects of smoking are akin to those of carrying an extra 100 pounds!

THE THREE MOST IMPORTANT FACTS YOU SHOULD REMEMBER

1. Excessive weight increases your chances for high blood pressure, heart disease, diabetes, cancer — all big killers. For recommended weight see Table 1.
2. Getting off the pounds makes a difference, both in the killer diseases and in how you feel on a day-to-day basis. An obese person who loses 30 to 40 pounds can make a huge difference in his or her medical picture. There may be important medical improvements in blood pressure, blood sugar levels, cholesterol and triglyceride levels, tolerance of exercise, medication use, hospitalization rate, days sick, and even mortality. And you'll probably find you're having less fatigue and more sex.
3. Excess pounds are usually put on slowly — five to 10 pounds per year. And they can be taken off the same way, simply by changing around

TABLE 1. Recommended Weight in Relation to Height

HEIGHT		MEN		WOMEN	
FEET	INCHES	AVERAGE	RANGE	AVERAGE	RANGE
4	10	—	—	102	92-119
4	11	—	—	104	94-122
5	0	—	—	107	96-125
5	1	—	—	110	99-128
5	2	123	112-141	113	102-131
5	3	127	115-144	116	105-134
5	4	130	118-148	120	108-138
5	5	133	121-152	123	111-142
5	6	136	124-156	128	114-146
5	7	140	128-161	132	118-150
5	8	145	132-166	136	122-154
5	9	149	136-170	140	126-158
5	10	153	140-174	144	130-163
5	11	158	144-179	148	134-168
6	0	162	148-184	152	138-173
6	1	166	152-189	—	—
6	2	171	156-194	—	—
6	3	176	160-199	—	—
6	4	181	164-204	—	—

Height without shoes, weight without clothes. (Courtesy of the Metropolitan Life Insurance Co.)

those eating habits that slowly put the pounds on and by exercising more.

How Much Should You Weigh?   There are a number of ways to determine this. Doctors grab a pinch of skin and see how much fat there is by how thick the fold of skin is. The easiest way is to look at yourself nude in the mirror, or compare a picture now with how you looked at graduation or on your wedding day or at some time when you felt especially happy and trim.

Or check your present weight and compare it with the table of desirable weights.

(Athletes often exceed these chart allowances but are not considered overweight. If you feel these charts are not appropriate for you, you may want to check it out with your physician.)

Note that the chart is for desirable weights rather than normal weights of the American people, which are much higher. Notice also that the ranges are very great—much depends on your body structure. Whether you use your past healthiest weight, the actual chart figure, or the chart with a little allowance for a heavy build, this gives a basic figure to work toward and tells you how far you have to go.

Why You Are Overweight.   After you determine how much overweight you are, the next step is to determine what the factors are that are causing you to be overweight. One study of overweight people who couldn't lose showed that they ate during emotional periods or at certain times by habit. Another study showed that when sandwiches were offered to thin people, they ate as much as they wanted and then stopped; obese people ate more sandwiches, as many as were put in front of them.

Test if you react to the following eating cues.

Do you react to stress by reaching for something to eat?

Do you eat as a way of getting back at someone else (see what you made me do)?

Does food give you a feeling of security and being loved, a feeling which goes back to childhood days?

Are you fearful of sex and find that being overweight sets up a protective barrier against being attractive?

Was food used as a reward or punishment in your childhood, and now you reward yourself and make yourself feel good by eating?

Do you often eat when upset, bored, lonely, or while watching television or reading?

Do you eat at certain times by habit, such as before going to bed or while watching television?

Do you eat just because food is available, eating whatever is offered to you whether you are satisfied with less or not?

Do you eat everything by habit because you learned as a child to clean
your plate, and you just keep doing it?

Do you eat whenever the clock says to whether you are hungry or not?

Can you pinpoint a specific time when you started gaining weight: as a
teenager, after you got married, after you got your job?

Did you discover that you suddenly gained 20 to 30 pounds in a year or
two, or did you gain a pound here, two pounds there, always creeping
up?

Are there certain high calorie foods or drinks that you have come to
regard as being important to you?

By thinking through these cultural and psychological factors that could be
influencing your eating, you can understand your specific problem better,
and so better design a plan that takes them into account.

Testing Your Calorie Balance. To do this, first determine accurately just
what you eat. Make a chart like the following one (Fig. 1) and on it write
in the actual amounts of things you ate today and what you ate yesterday.

Now for each food, calculate how many calories you took in. (See Table 3
on pages 130–132.)

List all foods and beverages, including snacks and sauces, and additions like
sugar, cream, catsup, mayonnaise.

What were your calorie counts?

Now rate yourself on this activity scale.

13   very inactive (a sedentary office worker)
14   slightly inactive (occasional games of golf or walks)
15   moderately active (frequent jogging, calisthenics, tennis)
16   highly active (almost always on the go, seldom sitting down or
      standing still)
17   very highly, strenuously active (a construction worker or other
      strenuous activity frequently)

Multiply your activity rating by your ideal weight to get the number of
calories you should be getting to maintain your recommended weight as seen
in the chart. A 200-pound office worker, for example, should be getting only
about 2,600 calories a day; a 200-pound athlete needs 3,400 calories.

If you are overweight and if you kept an accurate calorie count of daily
foods, you probably found your calorie intake was higher than your expenditure. The difference is what you need to change. (If you don't want to list
all your foods take your *present* weight and multiply it by your activity
number, and that will give you number of calories you are probably taking
in now.)

Remember in all these facts you are gathering, the purpose is not to judge
yourself, and not to feel guilty or defensive, but rather to look at the facts

FIGURE 1. **48-Hour Calorie and Carbohydrate Test**

DAY 1

Food	Calories	Carbohydrates (grams)
Breakfast:		
Lunch:		
Dinner:		
Snacks:		
Drinks:		
Total		

DAY 2

Food	Calories	Carbohydrates (grams)
Breakfast:		
Lunch:		
Dinner:		
Snacks:		
Drinks:		
Total		

119

objectively. Don't give answers with a feeling of self-incrimination, falling prey to the culture's game of placing blame. Don't think nonproductively of being a fat slob, having no willpower, or eating because you're mentally weak. Name-calling usually interferes with change and seldom contributes to it.

Step Three. Find Or Build Yourself A Supportive Environment

One of the greatest problems people have in losing weight and in maintaining weight loss is that they try to do it completely on their own. Tell your friends what you are trying to do so they will encourage you instead of trying to push fattening foods on you.

One of the primary possibilities for support in weight loss is your family. If everyone wants to lose, it's easy. If you are the only one who wants to lose, at least get the others to support you. Explain what you're going to do and just what will hinder or help you. This will make it easier for them to give you the support you need. (You need not go as far as one woman in a weight reduction program whose husband was undermining all her attempts to lose weight because he felt more secure when she was fat. She came to a meeting and announced she had lost 165 pounds all in one week — by kicking out her husband.)

Form a Lifegain group or join an already organized weight-reducing group as a simple way to be part of a culture that is predesigned to support weight loss. The weekly meetings in which an attitude of caring is generated and in which you are held accountable for your progress through weekly reports can be an important factor in treatment success for many people. The one problem is that these groups only meet weekly or monthly, so the support is not steady; however, they do help. Support groups that can help you every day are even more helpful.

Many of the same suggestions mentioned in the nutrition chapter apply here as well. Make sure, for example, that your pantry and refrigerator are nutritionally balanced — it's hard to reach over the cheesecake for the carrots.

Staying away from "occasions of sin" might help you. The authors once watched a group of people leaving a holistic lecture discussing where they would go to eat — it turned out to be the local sweet shop. Find substitutions for such places of temptation. Going for a walk can take the place of that hour in the sweet shop.

Get others on your side. Work out agreements with your family beforehand. Then there will be less chance of others' feeling hurt or deprived. With adequate warning, the family won't be critical of what you are doing.

Look at recipe books for low calorie dishes. A lot of people wouldn't mind cooking them if they knew how.

There are many different approaches and programs, varying from those in which you pay a great deal of attention to food weight, calories, etc., to those where you get your mind off food as much as possible. We are giving you some possibilities for plans, but there may be many others. The important thing is to provide yourself with a supportive environment. (There are a few weight reduction programs that need to be studiously avoided. Some liquid protein diets, for example, have had disastrous results for some people. Because there have been fatalities, any liquid protein diet should be adequately supervised by competent doctors.)

Objectives should be both short-range and long-range and should not be so extreme as to be impossible to achieve. Make the short-range goals easy to attain so in the beginning there is little chance of failing. The first successes will encourage you to continue.

The long-range objectives for a really large weight reduction should be spaced over a longer time—a year is a good target date. And with weight loss, your program is not really over until your ideal level has been *maintained*. Your really long-range objective: to stay slim for life.

Weight reduction can be carried out in many ways, from highly structured programs to very unstructured ones that require a minimum of attention.

MAKING THE DECISION

Now that you've analyzed your own weight, make the following decisions.

Check One:
- ☐ I am satisfied with my weight and do not want to change it.
- ☐ I think I would look better, feel better, and be healthier if I weighed less and so wish to lose weight.

The next decision to make after analyzing the data about yourself is what your basic problem is and what general approach is best.

Check One Or More Of The Following (You May Want To Do All Three):
- ☐ I think I eat too much and should generally cut down.
- ☐ I think I eat too many fattening foods and want to change the kinds of foods I eat.
- ☐ I think I am too inactive and want to exercise more.

Now Set Your Weight Goal:
- ☐ My present weight is ——.
- ☐ At the end of this year I would like to weigh ——.
- ☐ I have shared this with others and have taken the first step toward change. ——

Step Four. Some Alternatives That Work

There are many different approaches to weight reduction. Some possibilities that we have found helpful are listed below. For your convenience, they are placed in a week by week listing, but you should follow your own pace, and the final plan should be your own.

Since one key belief in Lifegain is freedom of choice, we suggest that you select your own activities and design your own plan, choosing from the options listed. The important thing is to be systematic and to use a step-by-step plan you believe in, building into it all the fun and positive elements you can.

Table 3 can be helpful to you in implementing your weight loss program.

WEEK 1. START THE BASIC LIFEGAIN WEIGHT-LOSS PLAN

To lose weight effectively, there are three basic things you must do, and you should start them right away.

1. Eliminate sugar, and food and drinks containing sugar as much as possible.
2. Eliminate refined carbohydrates (starches like pie, cake, cookies) as much as possible.
3. Gradually increase your exercise and activity.

There are two major approaches used in weight-loss programs: 1) reducing calories; or 2) reducing refined carbohydrates. Either is effective. Both together are even more effective. The Lifegain Weight-Loss Plan takes both into account.

There are a number of ways to carry out the basics. Look over the following options as you design your own action plan. They are ideas and activities that other people in the Lifegain program have found helpful. Mark off the choices that you think will be most effective for you and begin to put some of them into practice this week.

Start taking a brisk walk every day.

Learn to cook a low calorie gourmet dish.

Eliminate all ice cream, candy, cake, pie, jams, jellies, sweetened cereals, sugar on cereals. Drink water instead of sugar sodas. Eliminate the sugar in your coffee or tea.

Buy canned foods packed in their own juices or water instead of syrup or oil.

Don't eat any more cake or pie (one piece means about 250 calories) or drink milkshakes (421 calories).

Instead of bread stuffing, use vegetable or fruit stuffing or sprouts.

Instead of sherbet, use fresh fruit ice.

Instead of ice cream, eat yogurt.

If you serve hors d'oeuvres, use raw vegetables.

If you're going to a party, concentrate on protein foods and raw vegetables at the snack table.

Learn to eat the nonfattening way when you're out. Keep away from candies and pastries, concentrate on meats and salads. Eat the cheese wedge, leave the cracker. Eat the fruit cup, leave the syrup.

WEEK 2. SUPER WAYS TO MAKE IT EASY FOR YOURSELF

Keep up your basic three steps of eliminating sugar, eliminating starches, and brisk walking. They should be having some effect already.

A diet shouldn't be work, it should be fun. To make it easy, to make it positive instead of a denial, try some of the following.

Begin each meal with a nonfattening liquid just before you eat. Even a glass of water helps take the edge off appetite.

Cut down or eliminate your alcohol intake.

Don't put bowls of food on the table, so it becomes a special effort to get seconds.

Cut down drastically on fats such as lard, cooking oil, margarine, salad dressing.

Cut fat off meats. Substitute fish and poultry for some meats.

Use skim milk in place of whole milk.

Remind yourself with the words, "I choose to weigh less."

Carry a pocket calorie or carbohydrate counter with you and look foods up before you eat them.

Cut away the fat pads under the skin of poultry and game.

Broil or steam instead of fry.

Make broths, gravies, and sauces fat free. If you chill fat drippings and sauces after cooking, the fat will rise to the surface and solidify for easy removal. To remove fat while the broth is in the original pan, skim ice cubes through it.

Try a low calorie French dressing: Mix one cup of tomato juice and one-fourth cup vinegar or lemon juice. Add chopped onion, garlic, pepper, and any desired seasonings such as mustard, green pepper, celery seed, or bay leaf.

Buy only what is on your diet (what goes into your refrigerator goes into your stomach). By deciding to buy only what is low calorie and nutritious, you can resist the advertising efforts to get you to eat high profit foods.

Make a list of foods you ordinarily eat and determine which items you could cut back on to reduce calories or carbohydrates the most. Write beside each a less fattening substitute that you would enjoy.

Experiment with eating five small meals a day instead of three.

Reduce the amount of salt in your food.

Learn to enjoy food more: Eat more slowly, savor food, and enjoy the taste and texture.

Saute the low calorie way. Instead of using a lot of oil, use a heavy skillet and sprinkle with salt or just rub it with enough oil to prevent the food from burning.

Or buy a Chinese wok and do quick, lowfat oriental cooking.

Get rid of the calories you'll never miss. For breakfast eat a boiled egg (78 calories) instead of scrambled (120 calories), a slice of gluten bread (35 calories) instead of white bread (63 calories). Use skim milk (80 calories per glass) instead of whole milk (165); diet soda (2) instead of sugared (100). Instead of a chocolate malt (500 calories), have a lemonade with artificial sweetener or iced tea with lemon.

Instead of butter on toast (170 calories), use apple butter (90). Instead of cake (110), use cantaloupe (40). Instead of chocolate cake with icing (425), eat a bunch of grapes (65). Instead of fried oysters (400), eat them in the shell (100).

Try a behavior modification technique. When you desire a fattening food, conjure up an unpleasant thought until it wipes out the food thought, then shout "stop" to yourself to clear the bad thought. Now picture a nonfattening food and fuse it with a pleasant thought.

Separate eating from other activities; for example, don't eat and watch television, don't eat when you read.

Keep carrot sticks, celery, and other nonfattening food handy for snacks.

Paste a picture in the kitchen of yourself in a bathing suit at your current weight and another of you when you were slim.

Talk to yourself, making positive statements: "I won't eat this. I am going to be slim."

If you think psychological factors are behind most of your overeating, make an appointment with a psychologist or other counselor to discuss it.

Put leftovers away instantly.

When you feel hungry, take a shower, scrub the floor, call somebody on the phone.

Get yourself started in new activities. Get out of the kitchen. If your dates are usually going out to dinner, find another pleasure.

Break up some of your old habits. Have conversations in the bedroom or living room instead of the kitchen. Take a walk after dinner.

Try eating your biggest meal in the morning; your smallest meal at night. One family really liked this idea, thought it was an exciting way to beat a norm, and started getting up at 5:00 A.M. so they had time to have their family meal at breakfast. Then in the evening they had a light meal and had time for other family things: games, hikes, etc.

WEEK 3. GET SERIOUS ABOUT AN EXERCISE PROGRAM

When your expenditure of calories exceeds your intake, weight will come off, so use up calories through exercise in addition to decreasing your caloric intake through diet.

Opponents of exercise as weight reduction are fond of pointing out things such as "to lose a pound of fat you would have to bicycle for seven and one-half hours." But what they fail to point out is that if you cycled for one-half hour every day, you would lose a pound in two weeks. And if you did it every day for a year, that would be 26 pounds. Of course, this assumes that you add this to any exercise you already do and do not increase your caloric intake.

Most overweight patients have reduced lung capacity and inefficient breathing and heart action, so exercise at first may seem difficult. Start your exercise lightly and increase it gradually. How much you do will build up as you go along, because it will become easier as the pounds come off and as your capacity, skill, and conditioning improve.

The amount you eat and the amount you exercise have to balance out. Think of it this way: it takes only two minutes of swimming to counteract one-half cup of string beans, but 30 minutes of swimming to counteract 20 french fries; six minutes of jogging to counteract half a cantaloupe, but 42 minutes to counteract a chocolate shake.

Exercise does *more* than just use up calories. It helps speed up the burning of fats in the body, and it changes the level of insulin, a double-barreled shot for fat reduction.

Table 2, prepared by the University of Michigan and issued by the President's Council on Physical Fitness and Sports, will give you an idea of the comparative value of various activities in burning up calories to help you plan your own activity program. Try to pick activities you can do regularly. And don't forget walking. A good, brisk walk for 15 to 20 minutes daily can do wonders!

WEEK 4. IF YOU ARE HAVING TROUBLE LOSING

If you are not losing as much weight as you would like, don't put yourself down; simply read through the Lifegain program again to see if there are any essential steps you might be leaving out, if there are additional things among the options that you might do.

Be careful of medications that can be diet killers. Some medications can interfere with weight loss. Check with your doctor to determine if any medication you are taking could be the problem. Perhaps he can prescribe a substitute. And read the instructions inserted with the package to see if weight gain is listed as a possible side effect.

For many women one troublesome item may be estrogen, used to treat menopause or in birth control pills. If you are taking the pill and are overweight, ask your doctor if you can switch to a nonestrogen brand or to another form of contraceptive.

Some doctors believe that hormones injected into cattle to fatten them can prevent weight loss in humans. Try avoiding beef and see if you lose faster.

TABLE 2.   Energy Expenditure by a 150-Pound Person in Various Activities

ACTIVITY	GROSS ENERGY COST (Calories per hour)
A. Rest and Light Activity	50-200
Lying down or sleeping	80
Sitting	100
Driving an automobile	120
Standing	140
Domestic work	180
B. Moderate Activity	200-350
Bicycling (5½ mph)	210
Walking (2¼ mph)	210
Gardening	220
Canoeing (2½ mph)	230
Golf	250
Lawn mowing (power mower)	250
Bowling	270
Lawn mowing (hand mower)	270
Fencing	300
Rowboating (2½ mph)	300
Swimming (¼ mph)	300
Walking (3¾ mph)	300
Badminton	350
Horseback riding (trotting)	350
Square dancing	350
Volleyball	350
Roller skating	350
C. Vigorous Activity	over 350
Table tennis	360
Ditch digging (hand shovel)	400
Ice skating (10 mph)	400
Wood chopping or sawing	400
Tennis	420
Water skiing	480
Hill climbing (100 ft per hr)	490
Skiing (10 mph)	600
Squash and handball	600
Cycling (13 mph)	660
Scull rowing (race)	840
Running (10 mph)	900

If you drink, it may be the alcohol that keeps you from losing. One ounce of 100-proof spirits counts for about 20 grams of carbohydrates; or if you count calories, it contains about 100 calories per ounce. Sweet cocktails, sweet wines like sherry and port, and champagne are very high in both calories and carbohydrates.

Try high fiber bread. Studies at three universities have demonstrated the safety and effectiveness of this bread for weight control. An additional study with diabetic subjects has demonstrated the effectiveness of the high fiber bread and a high fiber diet in reducing blood sugar.

If you are severely overweight and are not succeeding in losing, go to a physician or clinic specializing in obesity.

If you use any fast action diets, be sure to still go through the basic steps of the Lifegain program to establish some support and the proper eating patterns, so you will be able to maintain that weight loss for the rest of your life.

Step Five. Keep Track And Tune In

Remember that one of the key steps in a change program is keeping track of achievements. It gives you a lift to see that something is being accomplished and increases your motivation for continuing.

Weigh yourself before you start the diet then weigh yourself at two-week intervals, weekly if you can't stand to wait. But don't overuse your scale since there will be temporary daily fluctuations, even fluctuations from morning to evening that will baffle you and might discourage you from continuing.

If you reach a temporary plateau, even if it lasts for several weeks, don't worry about it. It's typical. As long as you don't put on weight, you're doing all right. As you get closer to your target weight, the rate of loss will get slower.

If you just aren't making any progress, look over the action plan again to see if there are some essential steps you are leaving out or if there are some additional things you can do.

Other ways to measure progress: keep track of clothes sizes, belt notches, or body measurements (sometimes more accurate than a scale), or mark circles around each day on the calendar that you have stayed on your diet or kept below a certain calorie or carbohydrate count. It's also helpful to measure cultural changes. Look back over the Norm Indicator periodically to measure any changes in cultural norms of your groups, or just mentally check off changes that occur in your dieting friends or in support groups that you belong to. You will find a lot of encouraging examples of changing attitudes if you stay alert for them.

And tune in to how your body feels. In the first few days you may notice that you don't feel as well as you would like because your body is making adjustments, but even being aware of those will help you tune in to your body. Then in a few days, tuned in, you will see that the problems are gone and you will notice instead the surge of energy, the better coordination, the feeling of well-being, the fact that you're no longer carrying around that 50-pound suitcase. You'll find yourself looking in the mirror more often, you'll have a better image of yourself as a person, you'll find yourself expanding into other health areas that you didn't think were possible before, and you'll feel a new sense of power of what you can do in your life.

Step Six. Reward Yourself And Have Fun

Rewarding yourself is one good way of reinforcing your intentions. Remember that one of the reasons your culture influences you so much is that it rewards certain behaviors and punishes others. If you incorporate rewards for yourself as you achieve goals, you'll be reinforcing that behavior in yourself. Since you know yourself better than anybody else does, you should know what would motivate you the best.

Even very early in the game, motivate yourself by thinking about the benefits that will accrue to you as you lose weight as well as the reward you have decided for yourself.

Some people give themselves monetary rewards, putting aside a certain number of dollars for each pound lost and using it to buy something they really want, or they figure out how much the extra dessert or extra drink would have cost them and use that money for a gift for themselves. Some people imagine themselves thin and take pleasure from that image, even daydreaming of scenarios with themselves thin, or picturing themselves walking up a steep mountain without the 50-pound suitcase of extra weight they usually carry. Or they conjure up visions of the clothes they will wear, the comments they will get, the extra energy they will have. The images work, but the real sense of achievement is when you have actually reached your goal. Then give yourself a big tangible reward—you deserve it. Go buy a great looking outfit in your new size or whatever else you want to do.

Bonus: You may get a reward you didn't even expect. Many insurance companies give discounts on life or disability insurance to persons who maintain normal weight. One company gives about five percent off, depending on your age, if you don't smoke or are not overweight. For a free list of companies offering discounts, write Institute of Life Insurance, 277 Park Ave., New York, N.Y. 10017 with a self-addressed envelope.

Step Seven. Reaching Out To Others

As part of a systematic, overall change program, there are many ways to help and encourage other people and to support a positive culture to counterbalance the negative overweight culture. Give a real kiss instead of a candy kiss. Here are some other options to help you change those norms. Check off the ones that appeal to you, and alone or with a Lifegain or other group, try to put some of them into action.

If your supermarket has a section of food for weight-watchers, compliment the manager on it, and suggest it be expanded. If it doesn't have one, tell the manager you'd like to see it set up and talk with him about some ways he might make more money by focusing on low calorie foods.

Don't give high calorie gifts to your friends. Talk to the grocery manager about offering more foods without sugar.

If your school has candy machines, help the faculty and students think through if this is really what they want and if there might be better alternatives.

Wherever you find soda machines without juice or low calorie choices, suggest to the manager or owner that those choices be added.

Suggest to restaurants and bars that they offer low calorie food and drink; if they already have them, compliment them on it.

Protest television commercials and other advertising that push sugar and junk foods.

Compliment others who are trying to control weight and tell them how good they look if they have succeeded in losing.

When you have guests for dinner or have a party, always be sure your offerings include nonsweet, nonstarchy foods.

If you are giving a large catered party, have the waiters put nonalcoholic drinks on their trays so no one has to make a special deal of asking for them.

If it's difficult to buy nonsweet, nonstarch foods at coffee break or lunch time, bring your own; and don't hide it, show it off.

Suggest to your lunch group that you try a health food restaurant. And maybe you can get the group to take a walk or get other exercise during your noontime break.

If your favorite bar serves potato chips and pretzels, suggest some low calorie snacks. A bar in Sacramento, California, has started serving fresh vegetables—carrot sticks, celery, and zucchini. One of the bartenders explains it is by customer demand.

HOW TO FATPROOF YOUR BABY

- Don't gain more than you should during pregnancy.
- Breast feed. Babies who are breast fed are the least fat.
- If you bottle feed, don't insist your baby finish the bottle when he acts full.
- Don't start the baby on high calorie and high carbohydrate solids too soon.
- Buy baby food without sugar, or make your own baby food.
- Don't always keep your baby in a stroller. Let him creep, crawl, climb.

Does it work? Dr. J. C. Pisacano, of Long Beach, New York, reported at a meeting of the American Academy of Pediatrics that he tried a no-sugar, no-salt diet in 80 infants beginning at 3 months of age.

"We began to teach our mothers, the tastemakers of the next generation, the need to limit the amount of sugar in the diet," Dr. Pisacano said. "We held up for their scrutiny the contents of standard baby foods, dry cereals, popular snacks, drinks, and candies. We began to talk about making baby's food at home. We found great enthusiasm as we instructed mothers to add no sugar to the fruit they prepared, no salt to anything they prepared. Thus we effectively removed food additives, colorings, monosodium glutamate, and the unavoidable contaminants of commercial food preparation."

The results? By age three, only 1 percent of the diet group were overweight. In a control group fed the average American diet, 25 percent were overweight, the same figure often quoted as the average incidence of obesity in our American pediatric population.

The enthusiasm of the parents was so high, Dr. Pisacano said, that they asked to adapt the dietary regime for the rest of the family. It was a perfect example of how educating one person who sees results can then influence the eating habits of a surrounding culture — in this case the entire family.

TABLE 3. Handy Reference Calorie–Carbohydrate Tables

FOOD	APPROXIMATE CALORIES	CARBOHYDRATE (Grams)
Apple	100	20
Asparagus (1 cup)	15	6
Avocado (½ pear)	185	5
Banana (1 medium)	90	25
Beans, lima (½ cup)	100	17
Beans, green (½ cup)	25	4
Beef (hamburger)	300	0
(round 2 oz)	125	0
(sirloin, lean 3 oz)	250	0
Beer (8 oz)	120	8
Beet greens (½ cup)	30	2
Beets (½ cup)	50	7
Blackberries (½ cup)	50	14
Blueberries (½ cup)	45	11
Breads, cracked wheat (1 slice)	80	12
whole wheat (1 slice)	75	11
Broccoli (½ cup)	100	4
Brussels sprouts (½ cup)	50	6
Butter (1 T)	95	0.1
Cabbage (½ cup)	40	3
Cantaloupe (½ melon)	50	14
Carrots (½ cup)	25	5
Cauliflower (½ cup)	25	2
Caviar (1 T)	25	1
Celery (½ cup)	15	2
Cheese, American, Cheddar (1 oz.)	110	1
Cottage (½ cup)	150	3
Cream (2 T)	100	0.6
Chicken (½ medium broiler)	270	0
Cod steak (1 piece)	100	0

TABLE 3. (Continued)

FOOD	APPROXIMATE CALORIES	CARBOHYDRATE (Grams)
Corn (½ cup)	70	13
Cream (1 T)	100	1
Cucumber (½ medium)	10	4
Dates (1)	25	6
Egg (1 medium)	75	0.5
Eggplant (½ cup)	50	8
Endive (1 cup)	10	3
Escarole (1 cup)	10	3
Frankfurter (1)	125	0.7
Grapefruit (½ medium)	50	14
Grapefruit juice unsweetened (1 cup)	100	14
Grape nuts (¼ cup)	100	23
Grapes (½ cup)	75	10
Halibut (1 piece)	100	0
Ham, lean (1 slice)	265	0
Honey (1 T)	100	17
Kale (½ cup)	50	2
Lamb (1 slice)	100	1
Lemon juice (1 T)	5	1
Lettuce (2 lg leaves)	5	1
Liver (1 slice)	100	5
Liverwurst (2 oz)	130	1
Lobster (1 cup)	150	1
Margarine (1 T)	100	0.2
Milk, skim (1 cup)	85	12
Milk, whole (1 cup)	170	12
Mushrooms (½ cup)	10	1
Mustard greens (½ cup)	30	5
Oatmeal (1 cup)	140	25
Oil (1 T)	100	0
Okra (½ cup)	50	5
Olives (1 medium)	4	0.1
Onion (1 medium)	25	10
Orange (1 medium)	80	19
Orange juice (1 cup)	125	26
Oysters (5 medium)	100	3
Peaches, dried (½ cup)	100	60
Peaches, fresh (1 medium)	50	10
Peanut butter (1 T)	100	3
Pear, fresh (1 medium)	50	25
Peas (½ cup)	65	10
Pepper (1 medium)	20	3
Pork chop, lean (1 medium)	200	0
Potato chips (10 large)	100	10
Potato salad (½ cup)	200	15
Potatoes, sweet (½ medium)	100	18
Potatoes, white (1 medium)	100	21
Raisins (¼ cup)	90	28

TABLE 3. (Continued)

FOOD	APPROXIMATE CALORIES	CARBOHYDRATE (Grams)
Raspberries (½ cup)	45	10
Rice (½ cup)	75	29
Saccharine	0	0
Salad dressing (1 T)	25-100	1-4
Sauerkraut (½ cup)	15	3
Spinach (½ cup)	20	1
Strawberries (1 cup)	90	12
Sugar (1 cup)	800	194
Tangerine (1 medium)	60	10
Tomato juice (1 cup)	60	32
Tomatoes (½ cup)	25	5
Turkey, lean (1 slice)	100	0
Turnip greens (½ cup)	30	3
Veal (1 slice)	120	0
Watermelon (1 cup)	190	10
Wheat flakes (¾ cup)	100	90
Wheat germ (1 T)	25	7
Yogurt (8 oz.)	150	13

9 Drinking for the Thinking Person

Drinking alcohol has become an integral part of our culture. Think of the archeologists of the future trying to piece together our culture. The bars on every corner where people gather — a form of worship? Bottles of intoxicating potions of different flavors in nearly every home. Business gatherings, social gatherings of members of the tribe, usually centered around alcohol. Political leaders meeting and negotiating with it. Agreements made with clicks of glasses. Honored persons of the tribe given tribute by groups standing and raising glasses in the air. Toasts made at festive occasions. The customary tribal greeting: "Hi, come on in; what are you drinking?" Ingestion of the beverage as part of courtship procedures before mating. The intriguing names: Pink Lady, Orange Blossom, Stinger, Rusty Nail, Screwdriver, Goombay Smash, Zombie, Bloody Mary, Salty Dog.

Alcohol is the most widely used of our addictive drugs. And it's probably the one with the most confusion and myth surrounding it.

More than $250 million is spent per year advertising liquor. Americans spend $29 billion a year buying it. And the rate of consumption steadily increases.

The majority of people drink. Latest surveys indicate that in the United States two out of every three adults drink to some extent.

With the drinking culture, unfortunately, there often comes overdrinking. Then the grim facts reflect just how widespread the effects of the drinking patterns are.

For example, alcohol is involved in *half* of the highway fatalities annually in the United States, and the percentage is rising. (Alcoholics have a 45 percent greater chance of dying in a car accident than a nondrinker.) More than one-third of aviation accidents involve drinking; these are mostly in private planes.

One-third of sudden unexpected deaths among young adults are attributed to alcohol.

About half of all arrests are claimed to be related to alcohol.

And there are other risks when drinking in the drinking culture gets out of control: Alcoholics are absent from work about two and one-half times more frequently than the average worker. (Loss of production to American industry because of absenteeism, sickness, accident, impaired production due to alcohol is estimated at 10 billion dollars annually.)

And when drinking in the drinking culture becomes excessive, hundreds of thousands of families are affected; sometimes through generations, as the patterns are set up from parent to child.

It's the culture people meet every day in business and socially that encourages and supports an extensive drinking pattern, making it an expected part of most occasions.

And it's that same all-pervasive culture that usually starts people drinking. It certainly wasn't because it tasted good. Remember how a swallow of straight whiskey burned all the way down and brought tears to your eyes, and scotch tasted like the worst cough medicine you ever had?

But culture taught us it was supposed to be grown-up to like this taste, that the strange feeling was supposed to be pleasant, and that we were being clever and independent to defy and outwit the authorities by buying a drink before we were of legal age. We masked the rum with coke and tried to enjoy it.

Good times and friendship were associated with the drinks, and soon we really did enjoy it. We became acclimated, and then even the dizziness began to feel pleasant.

Now studies show that not just whether we drink, but also what we drink, when, and how often, are all influenced by our culture.

For instance, if you happen to live in the South Central region of the United States, you will likely consume less alcohol than those living in other areas; those in the Pacific and New England regions consume the most. If you happen to be an officer or enlisted man in the service, you will probably drink more than civilians. If you happen to live in a city or suburb, you will probably drink more than those in rural areas and small towns.

The highest proportion of drinkers, and the heaviest drinkers, are 18 to 24-year-old males. And the percentage of teenage drinkers is rising. Problem drinking is highest in dropouts and delinquents. Boys drink more than girls.

Why do people drink today? Because in our culture drinking is equated with sociability, relaxation, and pleasure. As part of the culture, people drink at parties and celebrations with relatives and friends. Children often see their parents happy and relaxed when they are drinking and therefore often think of drinking and pleasure together. And as we grow older, more and more are alcohol and pleasure mixed, until alcohol takes on the automatic association with pleasure — that's where the good times are.

But the problem isn't so much drinking; the problem is overdrinking. About one out of every 10 drinkers are problem drinkers or alcoholics. What makes the difference? We don't know.

But part of the problem is again the culture that says it's "big stuff" to be able to drink, it's manly to drink more, it's funny and cute to be drunk and to brag about it later, that it's a sign of a good host to ply everyone with many drinks.

THE CULTURE TRAP

It's the norm for some businessmen to have a drink or two before lunch, to meet after work for one or two more, or to have a few drinks when they come home after work to unwind.

It's the norm for people to push drinks on their guests when they give a party because they think everyone will have a better time.

It's the norm for people to think they can stop drinking any time they want, that they could never become addicted; that happens only to someone weaker.

It's these norms that often lead moderate drinkers into serious drinking problems and keeps them from making the change they want to make. If you're trying to change your drinking pattern and can't seem to do it, you should think in terms of what culture traps might be getting in your way.

THE LIFEGAIN PROGRAM FOR HANDLING ALCOHOL

Step One. Understand Your Own Culture

It's important to analyze your own culture and all those influences of the culture trap we've talked about.

Check over the following list to see what culture traps might be keeping you, or someone you know, from making an independent decision about drinking.

It is a norm in one or more groups that I belong to:
- [ ] for people to drink more alcohol than is good for them.
- [ ] for the host or hostess at a party to check repeatedly to make sure everyone's glass is full and drinks are being continually pushed.
- [ ] to persuade guests to stay for one more round or have one more for the road.
- [ ] to mention with pride one's ability to consume large amounts of alcohol.
- [ ] to have a drink when one doesn't really want to, just because the others are.
- [ ] for people who feel overburdened to seek relief through alcohol.
- [ ] for drinking contests to be considered an amusing entertainment.
- [ ] to consider drinking a sign of maturity and worldliness.
- [ ] for people to be offended by someone who refuses a drink.
- [ ] for people to drink more alcohol than is good for them every day or almost every day.
- [ ] to see alcohol as a necessary part of every social occasion.

☐   for people to think it's funny to see their friends intoxicated.

☐   for parents to consider drinking alcohol as proof of adult status.

Now that you think it through, how much do you think culture influences your drinking behavior? Test it out over the next two weeks. See how many examples you can identify in your group situations. Watch for these examples of cultural attitudes and norms at lunch, after work, at parties. Try *not* offering a drink when good friends come to visit and see how long you — or they — can refrain from mentioning it. Before you have that drink, pause for that millisecond — click — and make sure it's your own decision.

Step Two. Get The Facts And Separate Fact From Fiction

Bill was having drinks with friends at a bar near his office. He had started several months ago with a few drinks once in a while after work, and had recently added two martinis at lunch and a complete blast every Friday night after work. Drinking was becoming routine, almost a ritual. His wife was becoming increasingly worried and impatient. He was thinking maybe he should slow down a bit. He decided to head home after three quick martinis.

Driving down the expressway, he felt good; the alcohol had relaxed him, his future was looking rosy. He would really be able to start doing some good things for his family. But Bill never got to do them. His wife and two children waited at home in vain. They would never see their husband and father alive again. Bill was killed in a head-on collision. Two strangers in the other car died also.

That's the one big fact to know about alcohol: drink and you expose yourself to a possible death by violence. The biggest risk of drinking is that you might kill yourself or another in a car wreck, a fire, or other accident. In fact, one out of every four alcoholic persons dies by fire, poisoning, accident, or suicide. (The suicide rate of alcoholics is 58 times greater than that of nonalcoholics.)

The other biggest risk is that you may turn out to be one of the one-out-of-ten who gets hooked on alcohol, that the innocent drinking suddenly gets out of your control, affecting your job performance, your health, and your relationship with your family and others.

There are other facts you need to consider about alcohol too.

If you are a woman, you need to consider the fact that drinking during pregnancy can cause damage to the developing fetus (called fetal alcohol syndrome). An alcoholic mother in the throes of d.t.'s can give birth to a baby. Even the alcohol equivalent of two bottles of beer has been shown to cause a high concentration of alcohol in the fetus, 10 times higher than the amount found in the mother. One doctor found as many as 43 percent of babies born to alcoholic mothers had birth defects or died soon after birth.

You have to think of the potential damage that can be done to your body. The liver is damaged, and the damage is directly correlated to the amount of alcohol consumed. The first effect is a fatty liver — an accumulation of fat in the cells resulting in faulty liver function. It is usually reversible by withdrawal of alcohol, though suspected of sometimes causing sudden death. A more serious condition is hepatitis, an inflammatory reaction after alcoholic bouts, with severe pathological alterations in structure and function. The most serious condition is cirrhosis, a degeneration of liver tissue which is often fatal if drinking is not stopped. Drink a pint of liquor a day for 25 years and you have a 50-50 chance of severe cirrhosis of the liver.

Heavy drinkers also have an overwhelmingly higher incidence of high blood pressure, stomach and duodenal ulcers, asthma, diabetes, gout, strokes, pancreatic disease, and anemia. In addition, alcohol produces headaches, diarrhea, insomnia, irritability. Large doses frustrate male sexual performance by causing the liver to step up its destruction of testosterone, the male sex hormone; and it also causes long-term damage to the brain, researchers say. And now it is even being implicated as an added risk factor for certain kinds of cancers: cancers of the mouth, throat, larynx, esophagus, liver, and pancreas. (The risk is multiplied if you smoke.)

Most importantly, those who misuse alcohol tend not to enjoy life as much as they otherwise might. A walk after dinner is difficult when you've had too much to drink. So is sex, reading a favorite novel, or even having a pleasant conversation with family and friends.

Many people begin to drink to gain a level of relaxation in their free time and in their social relationships but end up drinking too much and thus impairing both.

Drinking for some people may not be harmful. In moderation it can improve circulation, lower blood pressure, and act as a mild and safe sedative. Some people claim that alcohol, when handled with care and moderation, seems to help them relax, socialize, and enjoy their meals more. We need to realize that even these enjoyments are culturally determined (Moslems, for example, would not consider these enjoyable), but when freely chosen they are less likely to end up interfering with our lives.

Whatever your choices, they need to be based on facts and some of these facts are not well enough understood by the people whose lives they affect.

FACTS BEHIND THE RUMORS BEHIND THE MYTHS ABOUT ALCOHOL

Check on these myths and rumors that are commonly believed in most cultures. Are they part of the belief system in your groups?

Myth. A person can never become an alcoholic if he or she only drinks beer or wine.

Fact. You can become an alcoholic on anything; it is a matter of whether you come to be dependent upon it. As one recovered alcoholic says, "I think most people probably believe as I did that you can't become an alcoholic drinking only beer. And yet, that's all I ever drank. I always thought alcoholism happened to the other guy and that I wasn't the type. And yet it did happen. Me, good ol' bright, middle-class Fred. I became an alcoholic on beer."

Myth. Alcohol is good for people if they are sick.

Fact. Not if you are taking medicines. Alcohol can react with cold remedies, antihistamines, tranquilizers, and sleeping pills to cause death. If you want to have a hot toddy with honey when you're catching a cold, do it alone, not with medicine.

Myth. A few drinks won't affect a person's ability to drive.

Fact. Alcohol first depresses judgment, next alters reaction time and vision, then attacks balance, perception, and coordination. Know how much you can handle and quit well before it's time to drive.

Myth. Women hardly ever become alcoholics.

Fact. Women in general drink less than men, but in the largest cities women alcoholics appear to match men one for one. In the rest of the country one in every five alcoholics is female. Women are often less noticed than men because they are less exposed to public view and often do their drinking at home.

Myth. You can't be an alcoholic if you never drink before 5:00 P.M.

Fact. It is not when one drinks, but how much and what effect is has that determines whether that person has a drinking problem.

Myth. It's rude to refuse a drink.

Fact. You can learn to politely refuse by requesting a different type of beverage. It is rude to try to push a drink on someone who doesn't want it or shouldn't have it.

Myth. Most alcoholics are found on skid row.

Fact. Less than 5 percent of the alcoholics are on skid row. And of the inhabitants of skid row, no more than 15 percent are alcoholics.

Myth. Some kids may be drinking a lot but at least they aren't on drugs.

Fact. Alcohol is a drug. It is classified as a brain depressant or anesthetic. And more and more kids are becoming addicted.

Myth. The heavy drinker must "hit bottom" before he can be helped.

Fact. The earlier help is given, the easier problem drinking can be helped. Sometimes it's just a matter of someone really caring.

Myth. Treating alcoholism is hopeless; the alcoholic always slips back.

Fact. Many alcoholics do have recurrences, but some two out of three do make it, successfully rehabilitating themselves.

Myth. People who drink too much only hurt themselves.

Fact. They also hurt their families, friends, employers, and strangers on the highway.

Myth. Black coffee, a cold shower, or breathing pure oxygen will sober you up.

Fact. Only time can sober you up. Although it depends on what you are drinking, as a general rule it takes as many hours as the number of drinks to sober you up completely.

But now let's look at facts about yourself. Remember to gather these facts in a nonjudgmental way, not putting yourself down and not becoming defensive either.

Many people with alcohol problems are "driven to drink" by their own tendencies to put themselves down. The best way to change behavior is not by attacking ourselves or calling ourselves weak. That only saps our energy, energy that needs to be put into positive action.

HOW TO TELL IF YOU COULD BE A PROBLEM DRINKER

It's important in making a decision about alcohol to be precisely and totally honest with yourself in appraising your present situation. Answer these questions thoughtfully and honestly.

Have you ever decided to stop drinking for a week or so but only lasted for a couple of days?	Yes	(No)
Do you resent the advice of others who try to get you to stop or cut down drinking?	Yes	No
Have you ever tried to control your drinking by switching from one kind of alcoholic drink to another?	Yes	No
Have you had a drink in the morning during the past year?	(Yes)	No
Do you envy people who can drink without getting into trouble?	(Yes)	No
Has your drinking impaired your family relationships, your work, your driving safety, or any other aspect of your life?	Yes	No
Do you ever try to get extra drinks at a party because you do not get enough?	Yes	No
Do you tell yourself you can stop drinking any time you want to, even though you keep getting drunk when you don't mean to?	(Yes)	No
During the past year have you missed days of work because of drinking?	Yes	(No)
Do you sometimes go on drinking binges?	Yes	No
Do you ever have blackouts during drinking?	(Yes)	No
Have you ever felt that your life would be better if you did not drink?	Yes	(No)

If you answer YES to *four* or more questions, chances are you have a serious drinking problem or may have one in the future. If you answered YES to any of the questions, particularly the last one, you may want to take this opportunity to begin to change things.

Or try this quiz from the National Institute on Alcohol Abuse and Alcoholism:

WHAT KIND OF A DRINKER ARE YOU?

☐ Do you think and talk about drinking often?

☐ Do you drink now more than you used to?

☐ Do you sometimes gulp drinks?

☐ Do you often take a drink to help you relax?

☐ Do you drink when you are alone?

☐ Do you sometimes forget what happened while you were drinking?

☐ Do you keep a bottle hidden somewhere — at home or work — for a quick pick-me-up?

☐ Do you need a drink to have fun?

☐ Do you ever start drinking without really thinking about it?

☐ Do you drink in the morning to relieve a hangover?

A social drinker should have three or fewer "yes" checks. Four or more "yes" checks do not necessarily mean you are an alcoholic or that you even have a serious drinking problem. But they should serve as real danger signals.

It may help you to keep an exact account for a week, marking the number of drinks, the size, and kind for each day on a card you keep in your wallet. You might also keep track of when your drinking caused any sort of problem, large or small, with your family, friends, work situation, etc.

As a further check, note the time and circumstances under which you drink. Does a pattern develop?

Watch for signs you may be drinking too much for relief of tensions and anxieties. In a study of 2,000 alcoholics, Dr. E. M. Jelinek found a predominant "prealcoholic symptomatic phase" which involved "relief drinking." Prior to drinking, the persons had been nervous, depressed, timid, tense, dull, or empty without knowing it or knowing what to do about it. Then, when they had a drink or two, they noticed that they felt better, relaxed, happier, courageous, free, alive, assertive, charming. In order to re-create these feelings, they begin to drink regularly. This does not necessarily describe all alcoholics, but it was found to be a common trait of the majority.

Step Three. Find And Build A Supportive Environment

Once you have made a decision to modify your drinking pattern, you need to find ways to communicate this decision openly and constructively and to build a supportive environment for the changes you contemplate.

The nature of your problem will decide you on the groups that you might consider becoming associated with. If your problem is a minor one, your Lifegain general support group or your own family and friends may be sufficient to get you through the changes you are considering.

If you have more serious problems, it is probably best to get in touch as soon as possible with one or more of the resources listed below.

Alcoholics Anonymous, P. O. Box 459, Grand Central Station, New York, N.Y. 10017. Check your telephone directory for local chapter. Members are men and women who have had problems with drinking and who help others. Thousands of chapters in 90 countries with some 800,000 members. Only requirement for membership is the desire to stop drinking. No dues. Free literature.

Al-Anon. P. O. Box 182, Madison Square Station, New York, N.Y. 10010. See telephone directory for local chapter. For relatives and friends of persons with alcohol problems. Group discussions and help with problems. Free literature.

Al-Ateens. Affiliated with Al-Anon. For children of alcoholics to help them understand their parents' problems, find support, and help.

National Clearinghouse for Alcohol Information. P. O. Box 2345, Rockville, Maryland 20852. Information on alcohol and how to cope with it. Literature, speakers, films for groups; aids to public and professionals.

National Council on Alcoholism. 2 Park Avenue South, New York, N.Y. 10016. More than 150 affiliated groups throughout the United States. Conducts informational programs for public and professionals, referral centers for guidance to those with alcohol problems, their families, and employers. Will give aid in establishing community or corporate rehabilitation and guidance programs. Free literature.

National Institute on Alcohol Abuse and Alcoholism. P. O. Box 2345, Rockville, Maryland 20852. The branch of the National Institute of Health that sets policy and programs to prevent, control, and treat alcohol abuse. Free literature.

Other places to check for treatment and counseling:

Company and union programs
State or county department of health, or commission on alcoholism, or mental health association
Hospitals
Mental health clinics
Church and religious organizations, clergymen

Many companies now have special employee counseling programs, and about half the employees using them are problem drinkers. If the employee accepts medically approved treatment, he or she receives the same benefits and insurance coverage as provided for other diseases. Job security or promotional opportunities are not jeopardized by request for diagnosis and treatment.

Veterans can receive treatment for alcohol problems at no charge. Treatment of acute intoxication is available at any V.A. hospital in the country. Many V.A. hospitals also offer comprehensive treatment and rehabilitation services for alcoholic patients.

Note: It is not necessary to become a complete and diagnosed alcoholic in order to gain help from these sources. Getting help early, when you're slightly dependent but need help, can be one of the best steps taken in preventive health care. The problem is easier to treat in its early stages, there is less likelihood that any permanent damage to one's health may have occurred, and early detection may help to preserve the family unit and your job.

MAKING THE DECISION

You now know some of the important facts about alcohol and you have analyzed your own drinking pattern and whether it causes problems or not. Now you can set objectives and make your plans.

It is time to make your decision. Your decision will be affected by the nature of the problem that you have identified. People who are alcoholics or who have severe drinking problems may need to get rid of alcohol completely. People who have minor problems may want to rearrange or moderate their drinking patterns to become less destructive or potentially destructive to themselves.

Check one of the following:

☐   I do not need or want to make any changes in my drinking pattern.

☐   I want to drink alcohol in moderation, but in control.

☐   I want to give up drinking alcohol completely.

☐   I have made my commitment openly to others.

☐   I have taken one step that shows my commitment in action.

Step Four. Put Your Plan Into Action

Your plan will be dependent upon the nature of the problem that you have identified. We have separated our suggestions roughly into two groups — serious problems of the middle and late stage alcoholic; lesser problems of the mild abuse and early stage alcoholic.

FOR SERIOUS PROBLEMS

If you have a severe problem with alcohol it is probably best that you look for help to the professional resources or Alcoholics Anonymous type support group programs that have just been listed.

You may also wish to consult with your doctor, or an alcohol information center in your area, an alcohol program at your company, or other program of your choice. Do it promptly and without embarrassment. The person you talk to will have helped hundreds of others already and may well have had an alcohol problem himself.

If you are a very heavy drinker, you may need a drying out period. Doctors call it detoxification. It's usually done in a hospital or residential center and is designed to get your body back to a normal nonalcoholic state without your suffering a great amount of d.t.'s and other withdrawal symptoms. Clinics used to give heavy fluids to counteract supposed dehydration of heavy drinkers, but recent evidence indicates most people during withdrawal are more likely to be *over*hydrated so this is usually no longer done. Cortisone is sometimes used to prevent d.t.'s. Sometimes tranquilizers or other drugs are used to help you get over this first difficult period. Antabuse is a deterrent agent (also called disulfiram) that, when taken regularly, causes a pounding headache, flushing, and nausea if it is followed by alcohol.

Nutrition and exercise are important for the rehabilitation of an alcoholic. Since alcohol has calories, heavy drinkers frequently substitute it for food and become undernourished. They therefore usually need extra vitamins. Sometimes vitamin B_{12} shots are prescribed, and other vitamins, plus calcium pantothenate, folic acid, and glutamine have been used as diet supplements. Frequent protein snacks have been found to help stabilize energy levels.

The professionals that you are working with will have suggestions on diet, or you may contact nutritionists in your area.

In the clinics emphasizing nutritional approaches, you will probably be given magnesium and large doses of vitamin B_6 to speed return to normal, and special diets will be employed.

A brisk walk or regular running will help the alcoholic substitute a positive "addiction" for the negative one and add to his or her general good health. The basic exercise program as outlined in Chapter 5 is a beneficial one to speed rehabilitation and help the body recover from the punishment it has undergone.

The Psychological Help You Will Get. This phase of treatment is geared to helping you recognize your problem, face it, and cope with it. If you are in a group you may see films, have discussions, hear others' problems and tricks they have learned. If there are family, business, or personal problems that have led to your heavy drinking, these are delved into and help is given in trying to solve them. When appropriate, family therapy sessions are held. Relaxation sessions may be used, behavior theory may be chosen, or transactional analysis may be applied. The purpose of all these sessions is to help you change your feelings and attitudes, face up to and understand the problems or influences that have pushed you to drink, and gain the self-esteem and confidence to stop your drinking.

FOR LESS SERIOUS PROBLEMS

If your problem is more a matter of being tied to some of the negative drinking patterns and negative drinking cultures that we have been describing, the ideas below may be helpful to you in developing your plan for constructive change.

You may wish to stop drinking completely, or you may wish to continue to drink but to do so in such a way that the actual and potential negative consequences can be avoided. Whichever you do, it is important that the culture be taken into account.

Controlling the Culture Traps. You know by now how important your culture is in helping you change or not change. So doing something about the culture you are a part of is a necessity if you are going to reach, and keep, your objective.

It isn't always easy to stay dry in a drinking world where alcohol plays a big part in the culture and lifestyle. Many of us live in the midst of an alcohol culture wherever we go — business lunches, conventions, holiday parties, every time we stop into someone's home for a social event.

Your only defense is to be constantly aware of the culture traps that are there waiting for you. "You're not drinking? — This is a party." *Click*. "Oh come on Harry, have one." *Click*. If you take a drink, make it *your* decision, not someone else's.

The nondrinking society leader simply drinks water at parties. "You'd be astonished at the number of people who are drinking water or soda rather than vodka at the posh parties. No one cares if you ask for a glass of soda."

One of your objectives must be to build the kind of cultural support that you need.

Some people find it most helpful to develop new interests as they reduce their use of alcohol. They get involved in some project that keeps them busy and satisfied. Some find it helps to avoid the bars and cocktail lounges where temptation is so strong; others find they still like the friendly atmosphere or music and simply order an orange juice or tonic.

One couple who decided to give up drinking completely said they found the A.A. philosophy excellent to follow. "The A.A. calls it the '24-hour plan.' We concentrate on keeping sober just the current 24 hours. We simply try to get through one day at a time without a drink. If we feel the urge for a drink, we neither yield nor resist. We merely put off taking that particular drink until *tomorrow* . . . If we are tempted to drink, and the temptation usually fades after the first few months, we ask ourselves whether the particular drink we have in mind would be worth all the consequences we have experienced from drinking in the past. We bear in mind that we are perfectly free to get drunk if we want to, that the choice between drinking and not drinking is entirely up to us."

If you are a mild abuser, you may want to consider some of these guidelines, following those that best fit your situation. (Caution: These do not apply to middle- or late-stage alcoholics who are unable to control drinking but must stop entirely. These people may misuse these suggestions, fooling themselves into believing that they aren't having a problem because they can follow them — or they rationalize that they are.)

1. Keep your daily consumption at one or two — well below the danger level of four drinks per day. (If you have high serum triglyceride levels, don't drink at all before checking with your doctor.)

2. Don't set up habits. Have dry days in between drinking days to give your liver a chance to recuperate and to assure yourself you can do without.

3. Pace yourself at parties. Don't bolt one drink after another. Sip instead of gulping. Put your glass down and concentrate on talking. If you're really thirsty, start out with a glass of water or fruit juice first. Between drinks have a soda with lemon or lime.

4. Know the tricks for slowing down effects of alcohol. Don't drink on an empty stomach. And while drinking keep sampling snack food, especially protein. Mix drinks with water, fruit juice, or noncarbonated mixes. (Carbonation causes faster absorption.)

5. Drink lower proof alcohol. (The proof number is twice the percentage — 90 proof whiskey is 45 percent alcohol.)

6. Don't get into drinking contests. It doesn't really prove you're a big man or a sophisticated lady.

7. Learn to judge your drinks. Your blood alcohol concentration is determined by how much you drink, how long a time you spread the drinks over, how much you weigh, how much and what type of food is in your stomach, your physical and emotional state. Alcohol affects women more if they are on birth control pills. A 120-pound beer drinker might reach the .10 percent intoxicating blood level with three bottles of beer, while the 180-pound drinker might consume five bottles to reach that blood level. Drinking martinis, a 120-pound drinker could reach the intoxicating level with one and one-half glasses.

   There is about the same alcoholic content (one-half ounce of pure alcohol) in a 12-ounce can of beer, a five-ounce glass of wine, the average cocktail, or a half of a martini. According to most estimates, your body gets rid of about one drink per hour by metabolism, perspiration, and urine.

8. Learn to watch for signs of beginning intoxication: slurred speech, numb nose, loss of balance when you stand up. Keep reminding yourself that you would genuinely be ashamed of getting drunk in public and losing control, that you want to retain judgment and reasoning at all times.

9. Don't drive if you've been drinking. If you are under the influence, don't drive, no matter what. Have someone else take you home, call a cab, or stay overnight.

   The National Highway Traffic Safety Administration and the United States Department of Transportation have prepared the chart (Table 1) to help you estimate by body weight how much you and others can drink and drive safely.

TABLE 1

BODY WEIGHT	DRINKS (TWO-HOUR PERIOD) (1½ ozs. 86 proof liquor or 12 ozs. beer)											
100	1	2	3	4	5	6	7	8	9	10	11	12
120	1	2	3	4	5	6	7	8	9	10	11	12
140	1	2	3	4	5	6	7	8	9	10	11	12
160	1	2	3	4	5	6	7	8	9	10	11	12
180	1	2	3	4	5	6	7	8	9	10	11	12
200	1	2	3	4	5	6	7	8	9	10	11	12
220	1	2	3	4	5	6	7	8	9	10	11	12
240	1	2	3	4	5	6	7	8	9	10	11	12

10. Be creative in dealing with your cultures. One couple who felt they were drinking too much decided to eliminate their predinner cocktails together but found that they really had lost one of the most pleasant parts of their day. They missed the sharing and conversation. They creatively decided they wanted the hour together, so they substituted nonalcoholic beverages with some super gourmet foods, music to listen to they had also been missing, and found their shared time was better than ever.

Another couple sometimes enjoyed alcohol, but at other times used a nonalcoholic relaxer: a hot bath when tired, iced tea instead of beer to cool off.

Others talked to friends they met with frequently and asked them whether they would be interested in drinking less at their get-togethers. Unexpectedly, the friends welcomed the chance to talk about it and said it would be a relief to get out of the drinking rut.

One man decided to spend less time with some neighbors who seemed to do nothing in their spare time but drink, and got involved with some new friends who spent their free time skiing and hiking.

Remember the warning signs that tell you that you may be developing a drinking problem. Some of the most important ones are:

- Gulping drinks to get the effect fast
- Starting the day with a drink
- Drinking alone to escape reality or boredom or loneliness
- Experiencing blackouts
- Drinking to relieve hangovers
- Having frequent minor accidents or other problems because of drinking

- Drinking with no dry days in between
- Drinking too much for relief of tensions and anxieties

If you are a pattern drinker, always drinking at a certain time or under certain circumstances, be especially alert and make a point to break up the pattern.

Living It Up Without Alcohol. And remember, not being drunk doesn't mean you have to be a wallflower. Live it up. Think of ways to have fun without alcohol. See if you can have a natural high just from your own good spirits and the camaraderie of those around you. Imagine how you feel when you have the "right" amount of alcohol and purposely act that way without it. Even experiment with losing your inhibitions and doing something silly and frivolous without a drink. If a party's so dull you need to have another drink to stand it, leave the party; see if that person in the corner also looking bored would like to take a walk and find something more fun to do.

Step Five. Keep Track And Tune In

Keep track of your progress toward your goals. Continue to note with interest but not criticism what times you want to drink and what times you don't and why. Also compare how you feel and function the next day after nights of no drinking or moderate drinking as compared to some of your prior experiences.

Think about how you felt before you started to change and how you feel now. Do you notice a difference in energy, alertness, concentration, fatigue, or even in how your muscles, eyes, and head feel? For people who are successful in changing their alcohol misuse patterns, the results will be immediately apparent.

You might want to jot down some of the good experiences that you are having now as a result of not misusing alcohol. Sometimes we overlook these and tend to focus on what we're missing instead of what we're gaining from the change.

After a month, think back over the last weeks and decide if you want to change your program in any way, and whether you are meeting the objectives you had set for yourself. If you are part of a group, talk over progress when you have the group together.

Step Six. Reward Yourself And Have Fun

You're probably saving a lot of money by cutting back or eliminating liquor costs. Put aside the money that you would be spending on alcohol and go out once a month and spend it on something special to reward yourself. You will probably be having a great deal more fun without the alcohol anyhow.

IS IT WORTH IT?

Singer–actor Kris Kristofferson, formerly a drinker, says, "I've got a lot more energy. I feel twenty years younger. There are a lot of fringe benefits to giving up liquor — less caloric intake and less getting in trouble. But I think the worst thing about it was the effect of the chemical on my brain and nervous system. I haven't been depressed since I gave it up."

Actor Jason Robards says his change was worth it. He decided to stop heavy drinking after a near-fatal automobile accident in 1972. "I serve wine and cocktails at home. I go into bars — love to be around drinkers — and stand up there with my coffee or cola or ginger ale on my own emotional high."

It is noticeable to friends, too. Betty Ford, when she declared she was beginning treatment for her dependence on alcohol and tranquilizers, found complete support and understanding from both friends and the press.

Step Seven. Reach Out To Others

Both drinkers and nondrinkers can be of great influence in culture change programs. There are several approaches you can become involved in, alone or with a group. Though you are only one person, you can become a change agent in your group, sparking a movement for a health change. If you get a group together and start building a moderate drinking or nondrinking sub-culture, you will find even more ways to influence the outer cultures. Here are some questions that suggest possible steps — any one of which can be an action that will help in some way as part of a total systematic change effort.

Does your local school have any educational program on the dangers of drinking and responsibilities of the drinker?

Does your company have a referral program for employees with alcohol problems?

Do you have friends with an alcohol problem who you think would benefit from reading about the Lifegain program?

Does your court system allow drunk drivers to accept treatment as an alternative to imprisonment?

Does your community have an alcoholism information and referral center to refer the person with a drinking problem to the right treatment resources? Check your local Community Welfare Council or Council of Social Agencies to see if your area has such a center. A "How to Organize" kit is available from the National Institute on Alcohol Abuse and Alcoholism.

ARE YOU A RESPONSIBLE HOST?

Part of reaching out is being the kind of host who does not act in a destructive way to his friends. In addition to what else we've told you, be sure to do the following:

- Stop serving alcohol about an hour before the party is to end. Bring out coffee and dessert or other snacks. They won't sober up your guests, but will give their bodies more time to absorb the alcohol they've already drunk for a safer drive home.
- If you see a guest who's drinking too much, offer to mix the next drink. Make if light and mix it with water or juice. Offer food that will slow down the rate at which his or her body is absorbing alcohol.
- Provide transportation or overnight accommodations for those unable to drive safely, recognizing that the host is just as responsible for preventing drunken driving as his guests.

Note: A recent court ruling has held that a host who has served drinks in his own home to a minor is liable for injuries sustained in an auto accident caused by that minor if inebriated. Tavern keepers are also responsible for "reasonably foreseeable" acts of a patron who has been served too much to drink.

IF YOU HAVE CHILDREN

Help your children to think through their own drinking cultures, about drinking behavior and responsibilities, and on the vital need to call you or a cab or to sleep over somewhere if intoxicated, rather than driving. If we can help our children think through the drinking culture, we can help them make mature independent decisions about alcohol for their own lives.

10

How Not To Be Accident Prone

You've heard of accident prone people; you may not have heard of an accident prone culture; but that is exactly what we have.

Accidents are the fourth leading cause of death today (after heart disease, cancer, and strokes). And they are one of the biggest killers and maimers of children. Some 23 million children under age 16 are seriously injured in accidents every year. For youths 15 to 24, about 70 percent of accidental deaths are due to cars or motorcycles.

Accidents are a big killer of old people too. Of all deaths from accidents, 25 percent happen to people age 65 and older, most often from falling.

More than 43 percent of accidental injuries occur in and around the home, with most deaths occurring from falls, fires, and poisonings. For every death from a home accident, some 150 disabling accidents occur.

Work accidents cost $17.8 billion a year, about one percent of our entire gross national product.

More than 50,000 people die each year in the United States from automobile accidents. This is about half of all accidental deaths and more than all the people who have died in major disasters of fires, floods, earthquakes, and tornadoes in the last 100 years! Another two million are injured annually in automobile accidents. Teenage drivers — both boys and girls — are considered to have about 90 percent chance of a crackup over a three-year period.

Almost half of all traffic accidents involve speeding or ignoring signals and warning signs. Drinking is also a factor, being involved in some 30,000 traffic deaths each year in 90 percent of all nighttime auto accidents. One expert estimates that at any average time, one out of every 50 drivers on the road is legally drunk. Drinking is also a major factor in pedestrian and home accidents. And more than half the people who die in swimming and boating accidents have high levels of alcohol in their bodies.

Why are we accident prone? Are safety practices really too much trouble? Do we just not think about it? Do we think the odds of being in an accident are so slight that we don't bother with the added safety factor? Don't we care if an accident happens to us? Or do we think that none of those bad things are ever going to happen to us. . . we're too invincible?

Sometimes people don't know what the proper safety precautions are. But most of the time they do know. Even people who go to the doctor regularly, get their shots, eat properly, and exercise frequently seem to ignore accident prevention as a way of increasing their lifespan and their enjoyment of life.

151

Most of the medical profession does not consider accident prevention a part of total health. But do broken bones, ruptured rib cages, fractured skulls have to have actually happened before we can deal with them as part of health? Must we wait until a person is bleeding in the emergency room before we consider safety a part of health care?

Somehow the public seems to feel remote from accidents. In one of the worst epidemic years, deaths from polio were only four percent of the deaths from accidents, yet millions of Americans contributed money and time to eradication of polio, while very little effort went into accident prevention.

For the major health improvement of the last 50 years, the simple increase in longevity, we can thank the Arab oil crisis because it reduced our driving speeds, which reduced the accidents.

One major reason that we don't think much about safety is that our culture doesn't encourage us to be safety-minded; in fact, it encourages us to take unnecessary risks. Some people try to judge cars for safety value when they buy, but it's hard to be objective when most advertisements stress speed and power more. Our schools teach children how to play soccer and football, but rarely how to ride their bikes or skateboards safely. We show our children movies of violence and thrills, but we don't teach them fundamentals about respect for their lives and the lives of others. We honor the risk takers in our society as heroes, even when their risk taking is foolish and without purpose.

A couple of years ago, in an attempt to cut the highway death toll, the Outdoor Advertising Association of America held a contest among advertising agencies to come up with a really effective safety message to get people to use their seat belts. The prize-winning slogan: "There's a name for people who don't use seat belts. STUPID!"

But it's not that we're stupid. It's that we are so deeply influenced by the negative culture that we do things contrary to our own best interests.

We are indoctrinated into an accident-prone culture from the time we are children. We play with thrill-taking super-hero toys. We hear men boast of danger and close calls. We see our parents take chances. We see society pay a million dollars to and make a national hero of a man who risks his life jumping a dangerous river canyon on a motorcycle.

The major use for CB's in cars is not for getting or giving assistance, but for getting reports on police to avoid being caught speeding.

To ignore safety becomes strongly identified with having courage. To meet danger, indeed to invite it and win, becomes a thrill. Seldom is thought given to the consequences if we should lose the encounter.

Think of seat belts. The experts have told us that only half as many people would be killed in traffic accidents if everyone routinely used seat belts. Yet only about 25 percent of us use them. In fact one survey, done just after a campaign on television bombarded people with the reason for using the belts, showed that 87 percent of the drivers in one town were cruising along nonchalantly with their belts still dangling by their sides.

The culture traps that encourage bad habits in smoking, drinking, eating, and exercise also prevail when it comes to taking precautions against accidents to ourselves and others.

In the scientific world that we live in, it is amazing how many people lose their lives through superstition. "If my number is up, my number is up." People don't often think of accidents as something they can plan against. We think of them as acts of God, completely uncontrollable, something that just happens. Sometimes we even look upon accidents as punishment for misdeeds or as undeserved blows dealt by a fate that is against us.

But you *can* develop a strategy against accidents happening to you, just as you can develop a strategy to reduce risk of heart disease or polio. You can develop a Lifegain Action Plan for safety just as you did for exercise, smoking, and eating, a plan to show what you can do to change your personal safety and your safety culture.

YOUR LIFEGAIN PROGRAM FOR IMPROVING YOUR ODDS

Step One. Understand Your Own Culture

Just as you analyzed your own culture for negative norms in regard to smoking, drinking, eating, and exercise, you can analyze your individual culture groups for attitudes toward accidents and safety.

Mark the statements that are true with a check.

It is a norm in one or more groups that I belong to:

☐   for people to drive over the posted speed limit.

☐   for people sometimes to be discourteous and unthoughtful of pedestrians and other drivers.

☐   for people to be concerned about their car meeting safety standards only at the time inspection is required.

☐   for people not to wear seat belts.

☐   for people to drive when drowsy or under the influence of alcohol or medication.

☐   for people to drive more rapidly than they should when there are bad weather or bad road conditions.

☐   for people to break safety rules and laws when they think they will not get caught.

☐   for people to sometimes use their automobiles as a means of expressing hostile emotional feelings.

☐   for people to leave pills and other dangerous or poisonous household materials around the house in easily accessible places.

☐   for people to look upon safety rules and regulations as something for others to follow — not themselves.

☐ for people not to use the safety equipment provided at work.

☐ for people to neglect the rules about how to operate equipment properly.

☐ for people to leave objects around where others can trip over them.

☐ for people to ignore safety violations or hazards rather than report them so that they can be corrected.

☐ for people to not bother checking on fire alarm and safety equipment.

☐ for people to consider having regular fire and other emergency drills unimportant.

☐ for people not to have any training in first aid and emergency procedures.

☐ for people to store flammable objects or chemicals near a stove or other heat source.

☐ for people to smoke in bed.

Once you're aware of the norms in your own cultures, you can choose to accept them or reject them. You can ask people who practice positive norms for support or choose to confront those with negative practices. And you can model — or demonstrate — positive safety norms to others. You can let people know you think safety is a matter of choice, not chance; that you're choosing safety, refusing to take unnecessary risks, not letting the culture control your thinking. You can let people know, "Around here, we think safety and think ahead, anticipating problems that could develop in the house or at work."

Step Two. Get The Facts And Separate Fact From Fiction

Now that you have analyzed the culture in relation to your own life, the next step is to analyze some of the myths about safety in our culture and then to analyze the safety practices you do or don't follow.

MYTHS ABOUT SAFETY YOU MIGHT BELIEVE

Myth. If you're a good driver, you don't have to worry about safety.

Fact. You still can't afford to speed or take unnecessary chances, because 50 percent of accidents are caused by the other guy. No matter how good a driver you are, if you're not in a position to slow down or stop when the other guy goofs, you are in danger yourself.

Myth. Accidents are a matter of fate and luck.

Fact. Accidents result from a sequence of events in which you, the way you feel, the physical conditions, and the culture all play a part.

Myth. You are most likely to be injured on your job than anywhere else.

Fact. Twice as many people are injured at home as at work and two and one-fourth times as many people are injured at home as in motor vehicles.

Myth. The accident death rate of the United States is about the same as that of other countries.

Fact. Our culture has a comparatively high accidental death rate. In Denmark, 11 fewer people per 100,000 die from accidents, and in England and Wales, the number is 17 fewer per 100,000.

Myth. It can never happen to me.

Fact. Why not? If there are thousands of fires in homes each day, what makes you think there won't be one at your house? If there are hundreds of thousands of accidents, what makes you think one couldn't happen to you? If there are thousands of drownings, what makes you think you are immune?

Myth. Safety rules are kid stuff.

Fact. They are kid stuff, since kids are frequently hurt; but they are also adult stuff because accidents affect them too, and what's more, their behavior affects children's behavior. You may have the visual acuity and experience to cross the street in the middle of the block, but your children may be watching.

Myth. Safety is nobody's business but your own.

Fact. Unfortunately most people who lose their own lives in accidents also take the lives of innocent victims.

Myth. If I haven't been in an accident so far, I probably won't be.

Fact. Statistically, whether you had an accident last week or not for 25 years, you still start from the same base each time you roll the dice or walk across the street.

Myth. It's "manly" and adult to take unnecessary risks.

Fact. It's one of the most immature things anyone — man or woman — can do. A mature person realizes he has a responsibility to others and has better judgment than to flaunt danger just to be cute or to show off.

Now let's turn to the facts about yourself and your safety practices.

Do you think you practice safety precautions as well as you could? Or do you feel it's easier not to have to think about it, or that it takes too much time to buckle the seat belt or put the guard on the equipment? Do you even consider it a boost to your ego to think you are above having an accident or that you are so courageous?

Check yourself on this quiz.

If you are involved in particularly dangerous leisure time pursuits (sky diving, motorcycle riding, scuba diving, etc.), have you checked out the hazards involved and done everything possible to reduce them?	Yes	No
Do you regularly check out possible hazards and dangerous practices that might exist within your home or work environment and take steps to correct them?	Yes	No
If you have children or young adults in your family, have you checked out the particular safety hazards of their activities such as swimming, skate boarding, bicycling, and driving?	Yes	No
When you are driving an automobile, do you consistently drive safely and at a safe speed?	Yes	No

Do you consistently wear seat belts or shoulder harnesses, even when driving for only a short distance?	Yes	No
Do you avoid driving when you have been drinking alcohol, taking drugs, or using medications that affect your reactions?	Yes	No
When you are riding with others, do you do everything possible to see that they drive safely and within the speed limits, or refuse to drive with them?	Yes	No
Do you avoid driving with others when they have been drinking alcohol, taking drugs, or using medications that affect their reactions?	Yes	No
Do you have a first aid kit in the house and car?	Yes	No
Has everyone in your family taken a course in first aid or studied a book on first aid?	Yes	No
Have you established what to do at home if there's a fire?	Yes	No

If you had all *yes* answers, your health practices in regard to safety are great. Keep them up.

If you had some *no* answers, you may be taking unnecessary risks, increasing your chances of killing yourself or others. You could mess up your life temporarily with pain, time in the hospital, losing time from work; you could mess up your life permanently (or that of others) by cutting off a hand, putting out an eye, scarring a face; you could cost yourself a lot of money (repairing damage, buying a new car, paying medical bills). You could also be a bad influence on others so that they practice bad safety measures and do any of the above to their lives.

You can reduce the chances of these things happening by reading the rest of this chapter and putting the many ideas into practice.

Step Three. Find And/Or Build Yourself A Supportive Environment

Since there are not many formal organized groups that you can join in relation to safety (although you might check your police department or the National Safety Council for local courses in defensive driving), the best way to give yourself some cultural support is to get your family, friends, or people at work to form a Lifegain group and work on safety changes together. Go over the analysis checklists, work on improvement projects, and meet occasionally to talk over how much progress you each have made.

One mother, shocked when a child was killed by running under a truck on a skateboard, got a group of parents and kids together in her house to look at what they could do to increase skateboard safety. The result: the kids built up their own safety programs.

Another group of people living on a lake became alarmed about motor boats. They got together to talk about it, then had the Coast Guard Auxiliary give boat safety and handling classes at the lake clubhouse.

Involving yourself with a group makes the changes easier.

MAKING THE DECISION

It is now time to decide what you want to do in your own life about accident prevention.

☐ I think my safety practices are already excellent.

☐ I think I'd like to improve my safety practices and improve my odds against injury or death.

My major areas that could especially use improvement are:

☐ car

☐ home

☐ job

☐ hobbies

☐ I have shared my concerns and commitment with others.

Step Four. Put Your Plan Into Action

The most important thing to do in setting up a new attitude toward accident prevention is to be aware of accident potential, to *think safety*. Remember, the whole point of the game is to get the odds in your favor. It's a gamble whether you have an accident or not, but it's a gamble you can have some control over. Even the simplest precautions, followed consistently, can shift the odds significantly in your favor.

There are three major things you can do about controlling your accident rate: be in charge of your own thinking (don't let your culture tell you it's good to be reckless); be on the watch and alert to what's happening to yourself (getting sleepy) or around you (driver coming out of the other lane, icy spots on the sidewalk); and think ahead (anticipate the things in the house your baby could get into, notice those kids playing on the side street near the intersection).

HOW TO INCREASE YOUR PERSONAL ALERTNESS WHETHER WORKING OR DRIVING

Analysis of accidents shows that there are 12 major factors behind most accidents. Look through the list and check off those that you are sometimes guilty of when doing a job.

☐ Being very tired or sleepy

☐ Being angry or emotionally upset

☐ Not having the proper skill for the job

☐ Having equipment in disrepair

☐ Daydreaming, not concentrating

☐ Being too young or too old for a job

☐ Being hungry, having a letdown feeling

☐ Being very hot or cold

☐ Working after drinking alcohol or taking a medication that makes you drowsy

☐ Working so fast you aren't safe

☐ Panicking in an emergency

☐ Taking chances

Then routinely be sure to do the things necessary to counteract those twelve factors:

Take breaks to prevent fatigue.

Eat snacks or take fructose or protein tablets to fight letdown.

Take time to calm down if you are tense, upset, or angry.

Don't rush.

Don't operate machines if you are very tired or don't feel well; don't drive or operate machinery or do dangerous jobs if you have been drinking or taking medication that makes you drowsy, dizzy, or high.

Vary routine to fight monotony.

Read instruction manuals, learn the proper and safe way to do things, get someone to show you if you don't understand how to work something.

Check equipment regularly, keep things properly maintained and neatly stored.

Don't show off, don't think an accident can't happen to you.

GIVE YOURSELF A SAFETY CHECKUP FOR YOUR HOME AND WORK ENVIRONMENT

Alone, or with your family or co-workers, go through this checklist for safety hazards. This is a great project to do with your kids—they love doing it and they learn something. Use a pencil when you go through the list and put an "X" by the questions you answer "no" so you will remember the hazards you find and will be able to go back and correct them.

In the kitchen and laundry:

☐ Do cooks in the family turn pot handles away from the front of the stove?

☐ Do family members know to slam down a pan lid to smother a grease fire, or throw on baking soda, but never to put water on a grease fire?

☐ Do you have a fire extinguisher?

☐ Do you have (and use) a little stepladder to reach heights rather than using chairs or boxes?

☐ Do you wipe up grease, food, or water immediately from the floor if spilled?

☐ Are chemicals and poisons stored in original containers, properly labeled, where children cannot get to them?

☐ Are insecticides or cleaning solutions stored where children can't get them?

☐ Are matches out of children's reach?

☐ Are you careful not to mix chlorine, ammonia, and other household cleaners which can sometimes produce a poison gas when mixed?

In the utility and work rooms:

☐ Are flammable liquids (gasoline, oil, paint, etc.) stored outside?

☐ Are papers and rags away from heat and electric equipment, including light bulbs?

☐ Are tools sharp and in good repair, stored in a safe place, unable to fall on anyone?

☐ Is the stepladder solid with all rungs and steps repaired?

☐ Are flues and chimneys working and unclogged?

☐ Have furnaces and heating appliances been inspected, cleaned, and adjusted by qualified personnel?

☐ Do the furnace and water heater have adequate air, with louvered door if they are in an enclosed space?

In the bathroom:

☐ Are medicines where children can't get at them?

☐ Are there carpets in the bathroom to prevent slipping?

☐ Are all electric appliances away from water?

Throughout the house:

☐ Are toys and other things put away so they won't be tripped over?

☐ Are screens securely fastened and windows locked or protected so small children can't fall out?

☐ Do stairs have a handrail?

☐ Is lighting on stairways bright enough?

☐ Can lights be turned on from both the top and bottom of the stairs?

☐ Are stairs free of clutter?

☐ Do large glass areas have furniture or planters in front of them, or decals so people won't walk through the glass?

☐ Are any wires frayed or cracked? Are there any electric cords running through door jambs or anywhere else where they are exposed to constant chafing?

☐ Are space heaters the type that don't tip easily?

☐ If you have a gas heater, is it properly exhausted and does it get enough fresh air?

☐ Do you have a smoke detector?

Outside:

☐ Are paths and sidewalks clear?

☐ Are porches, railings, and steps in good repair?

☐ Do grasscutters know not to cut the lawn when the grass is wet and slippery?

☐ Do children know about the dangers of running into streets?

☐ Do they know not to stand near swings?

Hobbies and sports:

☐ Are guns, bows and arrows, darts, and slings put away where children can't reach them? Do they know they should only be used with adult supervision?

☐ Do hunters in the family know to treat every gun as if it were loaded, keeping the muzzle pointed in a safe direction? To never load a gun unless intending to shoot it at something? To keep the safety on? To open bolts when leaving guns unattended?

Machinery and special equipment at work and at home:

☐ Do persons know to keep safeties, guards, and shields in place on machinery?

☐ Do they always shut off the power when adjusting, servicing, or unclogging machines?

☐ Do they know not to let machines run unattended?

☐ Do they know to shut off the motor when leaving a job temporarily?

☐ Do they know not to refuel hot or running engines?

☐ Do they know not to smoke when refueling?

☐ Do children know to keep away from machines?

☐ On hazardous jobs, does everyone know not to wear loose clothing?

☐ Is everyone careful to read labels on chemicals, to follow the directions, to use protective gloves and glasses when needed, to ensure good ventilation when working with toxic fumes?

☐ Is everyone careful not to burn discarded chemical containers and not to pour chemicals on the ground or into a stream?

Now go back over the analysis you did, looking at the items you checked off that need correction, and actually start to work on at least one of them this coming afternoon or evening. Alone, or with family and co-workers, work on several items each day.

THE LIFEGAIN ACTION PLAN FOR DRIVING SAFETY

Just because your license hasn't been revoked or you haven't been arrested doesn't mean you are a good driver. Try taking this quiz and judge how good you really are.

☐ Is my car inspected and in good operating condition?

☐ Do I periodically check safety devices — brakes, horn, windshield wipers, lights, turn signals, exhaust system — to see that they are working properly?

☐ Do I carry at least the minimum legal insurance?

☐ Do I use my seat belt *all* the time?

☐ Do I insist that my passengers use their seat belts?

☐ Do I abide by posted speed limits and other traffic regulations?

☐ Do I practice courtesy toward other drivers and pedestrians rather than trying to beat them out?

☐ Do I wait for an hour to drive after I have been drinking?

☐ Do I avoid driving if I am taking a medication that makes me drowsy, dizzy, or high?

☐ Do I avoid driving when I am very tired or ill or furiously angry?

☐ Do I really concentrate on the road and avoid daydreaming while driving?

☐ Do I pull over to the side and stop instead of trying to read directions or check a map while driving?

☐ Do I know: never to run an automobile in an enclosed space, even for a few minutes; to shut off the engine if I sit in a parked car for more than a few minutes unless the windows are open; to keep the exhaust system in good repair?

Your answers should all be yes. Questions you answered no to suggest an area that could be a danger to you and those who ride with you.

Consider how little it takes to cause an accident and how little effort it takes to prevent one. Judge for yourself whether or not you are as good a driver as you would like to be.

Then put a plan into action.

Make sure all the safety devices in your car work properly — brakes, horn, windshield wipers, lights, turn signals. If any is out of order, have it fixed.

If you don't already wear a seat belt, start today. Remember that you can cut your chances of being fatally injured in an auto accident by one-half just by wearing your seat belt.

Insist that your passengers also wear seat belts. (While they are riding in your car, their lives are in your hands, and to change the culture you have to constructively confront behavior that is dangerous to your — or others' — health.)

Obey the speed limits and other traffic regulations. Drive more slowly at night and in bad weather. Don't tailgate, it's a number-one killer (allow a car length for every 10 miles of speed). Don't weave from lane to lane.

Drive defensively — the other fellow may be drunk or incompetent. Watch ahead for possible hazards.

Don't drink or take medicines that bother you when you drive.

Support good driving habits in those at home, and at work. See that your spouse, children, parents, friends, all drive safely.

A PLAN FOR PARENTS — 14 UNBREAKABLE RULES FOR PARENTS OF BABIES AND YOUNG CHILDREN

Never leave your baby or preschool child alone in the house.

Never leave a baby alone on anything from which it could fall.

Always keep the sides of the crib up when not holding a baby.

Never leave a baby alone in the tub, even for a second.

Keep tiny swallowable objects — pins, buttons, beads, pebbles — out of reach.

Keep medicines, poisons, household cleaners well out of reach or locked away.

Teach your children to not eat plants or berries. Many common plants are poisonous.

Never allow a child to play in or near a driveway or garage.

Keep matches in containers completely inaccessible to young children.

Always stay with your child near water. Be sure pools, wells, and cisterns are protected.

Equip upstairs windows with sturdy screens and guards. Use gates at the top and bottom of stairs until the child handles stairs well.

Be sure there is no peeling paint on walls, windows, or window sills. Eating only a few chips can give serious lead poisoning.

Keep knives and sharp objects stored away.

Always use an approved car seat.

Teach your child about safety. Preschoolers need simple clear safety rules: Stay out of the street. No playing in the driveway. Sit quietly in the car. Never play with matches. Don't put tiny things like coins or marbles in your mouth. Hold someone's hand when crossing the street.

Don't just tell them, but show them and talk it over with them so they see how much they have learned. Don't have too many rules but be consistent about them.

As they prove that they have learned the rules, reward them. When Alice learns not to climb around in the car, compliment her. "Now that I can trust you in the car, I'll take you on a trip to the zoo."

And most important for a parent, show your children a good example. They are going to model themselves after you in attitude and action.

For example, to prevent inhaling a foreign body, the single most common cause of accidental deaths in the home among children under six years of age, the American Lung Association recommends that you never give peanuts, hard candy, or foods with small bones or seeds to young children; that you inspect your baby's toys for small loose parts such as eyes or buttons; that you don't let babies play on the floor until it has been cleared of all small objects they might put in their mouths; and that you encourage your child to eat slowly and chew his food thoroughly. They also stress that it is important not to set a bad example for children by holding pins or other small objects in your mouth or biting pencils, toothpicks, or straws.

CHECK YOURSELF OUT FOR SAFETY IN SPORTS

Whether it's the sea, the air, guns, or mountains you are involved with, show the proper respect. The one who is calm, cool, and follows safety rules is the truly sophisticated sportsperson, no matter what the person's age.

Check out these fundamental safety measures for ones that pertain to your sport and make sure that you follow them.

If you're in the sun, get your suntan gradually. The best lotion to prevent sunburn is PABA (paraaminobenzoic acid) in alcohol. If you are very sensitive to the sun, you can obtain protection with PABA pills or with Solatene, a new pill containing beta-carotene, both available in drugstores without prescription.

If you are out in extreme cold, dress warmly, stay dry, don't stay out for a long time, and watch for severe fatigue or parts that look white, gray, tingle, or have no feeling. It means frostbite.

If you are allergic to insects, help keep them away by taking a vitamin B_1 capsule before you go out (the odor appears on the skin) and use a repellant. If you are very allergic, carry antihistamine and adrenalin with you.

If you hike or climb, wear high leather boots to protect your ankles in snake country. Look before you step or put your hands anywhere.

If you're a skier, tennis player, or other highly exertive sportsperson, do muscle-strengthening exercises before the season starts and take professional lessons to avoid accidents. (They most often happen to novices.)

If you swim, learn to be a good swimmer. Don't go swimming after you eat or when you are tired. If you get cramps, don't panic or thrash around but tread water with your arms or float, and take deep breaths of air.

If you skin dive, don't try to establish records for time or distance, don't wear white or flashy bathing suits or jewelry that attract sharks and barracuda, avoid caves, don't dive where fish are being caught by boaters, avoid heavy boating areas, remove speared fish from the water. Always dive with a buddy.

BIKE RIDER'S SAFETY RULES

- Observe all traffic regulations — red and green lights, one-way streets, and stop signs.
- Keep to the right and ride in a single file.
- Have a white light in front and a reflector on the rear for night riding.
- Wear white or light-colored clothes at night.
- Have a bell or horn and use it.
- Always ride at a safe speed and be in complete control.
- Give pedestrians the right of way.
- Look out for cars pulling out into traffic from curbs and driveways.
- Keep a sharp lookout for sudden opening of doors on parked cars.
- Ride in a straight line. Do not weave in or out of traffic or swerve from side to side.

- Always use proper hand signals for turning and stopping.
- Slow down at all intersections and look to the right and left before crossing. (Some 80 percent of all bicycle deaths are linked to improper crossing of a roadway or darting into a road.)
- Never carry other riders. Carry no packages that obstruct vision or prevent control.
- Never hitch on other vehicles.
- Keep your bicycle in good running condition.
- Park your bicycle in a safe place where no one will fall over it.

Step Five. Keep Track And Tune In

You can keep track of your results on a formal or informal basis. Set a specific time, say in one week, and then both at home and at work go over the lists again to see how much progress you have made toward your goals. Then you can start concentrating further on the areas that still need work until you feel satisfied that you have succeeded in changing the things you wanted to change. Do these checkups periodically.

Tune in to yourself occasionally to see how many old tapes are playing in your head that are keeping you from safety. . . the show-off tape, the it's fate tape. Tune in to your own life wish and your concern for other people. Tune in your ability to get other people to think about protecting themselves. A discussion with a friend about seat belts might be better than sending flowers to the funeral.

And tune in to how much more you feel a part of your environment when you practice safety rules. If you're on the sea and practicing safety rules, it makes you in tune with the sea; you're not daring it, you're respecting it. The sailors who are good are in tune with the sea; the ones who are not, frequently are dead.

Another excellent ongoing technique: Every time someone in your family has a minor accident or a close call, as soon as possible sit down with everyone and analyze what happened. Avoiding accidents is your goal, but when they do occur, or almost occur, you can learn a lot by thinking about what could have been done to prevent it. And this is another time to be nonjudgmental. Instead of screaming at your child, or becoming hysterical, if he runs into the street and almost gets hit by a car, use the opportunity to make him realize that very real dangers exist.

Step Six. Reward Yourself And Have Fun

There are a lot of fun things to do that aren't dangerous, but if you choose to do things that are dangerous, take the precautions necessary.

One reward you will certainly have for having adopted safety practices and attitudes at home, at work, and in your hobbies will be the knowledge that you have acted responsibly toward yourself and others, which could have lifelong influences on your life and theirs. When you practice safety, you become a better driver, a better sailor. As you learn more about your hobby or sport, you acquire new skills and can now feel more self-confident and enjoy it more. You're now a better driver or a better boatsman or a more competent craftsman, and because you're more skilled, you also have more fun. Give yourself the credit you deserve, and more than that, buy yourself something to reward yourself. Relate it to where you have put in the most effort at safety; perhaps new cushions for your boat, rear speakers or new floor mats for your car, a new tool, new curtains for the kitchen.

Step Seven. Reach Out To Others

By emphasizing a positive concern for another person we are expressing our love for them.

Supporting good safety practices in others is a deeper mark of friendship than visiting them in the hospital after they've been hurt.

Help your spouse, parents, and children examine their own safety habits. When your child gets his first bicycle, or even a tricycle, help him to think through where he can and cannot ride, and teach safety procedures and respect for those walking.

See that your children know the dangers of skateboards and motorbikes.

Teach your children safe handling of tools and equipment and help them see what they can do about making their day-to-day activities safer.

See that your child learns how to swim, and swim well. It's not a matter of recreation, it can be a matter of life and death.

At work, encourage your co-workers to practice safety, and support them in following company safety regulations.

In some cases it is necessary to confront people who are endangering their lives or the lives of others. When you do so, do it in a nonhostile way. For example, if you are driving with someone who is going too fast, tell them you are really concerned about the speed at which they are driving and you would really appreciate it if they slowed down.

Check your community's safety practices. If you note a highway hazard such as a bush blocking the view of traffic at an intersection, a tree blocking a sign, or other dangers, report it, preferably in writing to your local police department. Is there a plan for emergency disasters? Is there adequate ambulance equipment? Are there lifeguards at beaches or pools?

Involve others in your community in a cultural change effort. The safety hazards you observe can be more readily changed with wider support, and the general raising of safety consciousness will be a gratifying outcome of your joint efforts.

SUPPORT MATERIALS

A number of agencies have excellent materials available, much of it free, that you can use to get safety education programs started or improved at your local schools, in your family, at the office, in the shop. Here are some of them:

Metropolitan Life, 1 Madison Avenue, New York, New York 10010. Films for free loan, brochures free for individual use or for quantity use in school, colleges, community groups, business. Provides help with program planning. Special material: safety guide for baby sitters, potential accidents for children of different ages, your health and driving.

National Safety Council, 425 N. Michigan Avenue, Chicago, Illinois 60611. Special detailed manuals and safety packages for industries of all sizes, including trucking and hospitals; newsletters for specialized fields from aerospace to wood products; films for school, business, and community. Hundreds of posters, signs, labels, banners, and other products. Safety training institutes, home study courses. Brochures on bicycle safety, home safety, farm safety, driving safety. Defensive driving courses. A 72 page directory lists all services. Reasonable prices for quantity material.

National Institute for Occupational Safety and Health, 4676 Columbia Parkway, Cincinnati, Ohio 45226. Detailed health and safety guides for nearly every specific business and industry of all sizes from auto repair shops to foundries, hotels, and bakeries. No matter what business you are in, this agency has material to analyze the hazards of that business and how to cope with them. Their list of publications will give you excellent ideas for things to order to decrease hazards at your job.

Bicycle Manufacturers Association of America, 1101 15th Street, N.W., Washington, D.C. 20005. Bicycle safety materials, including a bike safety kit available in quantity to educational and community groups.

Office of Child Development. U.S. Department of Health, Education and Welfare, Superintendent of Documents, United States Government Printing Office, Washington, D.C. 20402. *Safe Toys for Your Child*, *Pocket Guide to Baby-sitting*, and other health and safety brochures. Single copies are free.

United States Consumer Product Safety Commission, Washington, D.C. 20207. Fact sheets on product safety, industry toys, bicycles, playground equipment, ovens, televisions sets, flammable fabrics. Toll-free number: 800-638-2666.

11 Living Relaxed

From the moment of birth most of us live our lives encapsulated in a stress-laden culture. We are pushed and pummeled through the birth canal, startled by bright light, held dangling by our feet while we flail the nonsupporting emptiness of air. And sometimes our environment seems to fill our lives with physical and emotional stress ever after.

Our world is overcrowded and yet we are increasingly isolated from each other. Our cities teem with people — and loneliness. Our streets are clogged with traffic, our cities are dirty; our countrysides littered and noisy. We read of violence and drugs and pollution; of overpopulation and dangerously depleted natural resources; of the extinction of whales and the bludgeoning of 100,000 dolphins in blood reddened waters; of wars and kidnappings and terrorists and the seething unrest swelling through the land.

Stress builds.

And it builds more, as we are loaded constantly with change.

We no longer spend long periods in one neighborhood, at one occupation, or with one spouse. In our 70 largest cities, people move once every four years. We constantly encounter new people, new problems, new adjustments, more stress. Each change requires us to cope with more decisions and more new things to get used to. The decisions often make many of us anxious, pressured, and overwhelmed with the new.

It overloads our brains and our circuits always seem busy. Buffeted by the turbulence; bombarded by the noise and the crowds and the decisions; called on for action, action, action, we are all living in Alvin Toffler's *Future Shock*. But the future is now.

We live in a "pressure cooker," in a culture undergoing rapid change, making us cope with tomorrow today.

Constant tension has become the norm. We expect it. We admire those who seem to thrive on pressure. We reward each other for superhuman efforts. We set out to make it to the top and often push ourselves to the breaking point.

As the pressures relentlessly mount, little problems seem huge: tension, irritability, and anger grow.

Even when we try to relax, we sometimes can't. We go away on vacation, but it often takes such planning and costs so much we come back exhausted. Television programs, watched for relaxation, key us up with excitement and violence.

And though there are simple techniques for relaxation available (and a growing awareness of them) many of us still do not take advantage of them. Biofeedback seems strange and "far out;" meditation is "Eastern nonsense" or "OK for the yogis of India, but has nothing to do with me." Because we are medically oriented, we rely on the medicines and prescribed drugs which are helpful and even necessary in crisis times, but which might not be needed if we practiced preventive medicine more and tuned in to our bodies' needs.

In short, there are four ways our stress culture affects us: It provides us with a highly charged environment; it causes us to see that environment as inviolate and unchangeable; it influences us to respond to that environment in ways that get further in the way of relaxation; and it cuts us off from some simple stress-reducing techniques that would be of great benefit.

The sum total of these four aspects of our stress culture is that we are not enjoying life as fully as we could. The stress culture not only shortens our lives but decreases the quality of the years that we have left. It's high time we understood it and began to deal with it. It's high time we began to build more relaxing environments.

JUST WHAT IS STRESS?

What is stress really? Some people use the word stress to mean the situation causing tension. Others use the term to refer to the reaction to a situation; they call the situation a stressor. Stress, they say, is your body's survival mechanism. It's what made the caveman run or fight furiously when a saber-toothed tiger walked into his cave.

The way it works: In a stressor situation our glands pour out adrenalin and other hormones which quickly flood our bodies and set up an automatic "fight or flight" response. Our hearts beat faster, our lungs speed up breathing, our blood sugar level goes up, our digestion slows, and blood surges to our tensing muscles ready to act. In a life-threatening situation we can perform mental and physical feats not possible under ordinary circumstances.

The reaction can save our lives or give us the strength to save someone else's.

Today the "fight or flight" response is often brought on in situations that require us neither to fight nor to flee. And when this happens repeatedly, we have bodily changes that can cause great trouble, even bring on a heart attack or stroke.

Sometimes there appears to be no way to reduce stress. The problem isn't as simple as confronting a saber-toothed tiger. It's often a complex, insurmountable problem seemingly out of our control.

When the stress situation isn't resolved or keeps recurring so there is constant tension, your motor continues to race, your alarm button doesn't turn off. Your body is kept in a constant state of increased blood pressure, heart rate, and body metabolism. You scream at the children, swear at the slow traffic, go tensely through your job. The blood pressure goes up and stays up, a condition we call hypertension.

Hypertension is called the silent killer because it comes without warning, usually producing no pain or other symptoms before causing strokes, heart attacks, or severe damage to body organs. This happens because consistently high blood pressure causes blood clots, calcium, and fats to collect within the walls of the arteries, making them more rigid and partially or completely blocking the blood flow.

Sometimes there is a discernible reason for hypertension—pregnancy, childbirth, or tumors—but in over 90 percent of the cases, there is no specific cause. When there is none, we call it "essential hypertension," and the generally accepted cause is stress.

Evidence that stressful situations do cause problems for people has been proven in numerous studies. For example, one study of air traffic controllers found they had four times more high blood pressure and twice the rate of ulcers and diabetes as a comparable group of workers with similar medical and physical backgrounds who worked under less stressful conditions.

A study of employees at the Kennedy Space Center suggests that working under constant threat of unemployment was a major factor in the deaths of a group of young men with an average age of 31 who died of heart attacks.

People react to stress in very different ways.

Some people can handle the stressors of deadlines and big decision but not the inner stress of insecurity, inadequacy, loneliness, boredom, frustration, and not having control over one's life.

Some are always keyed up, tense, waiting for the worst possible thing to happen when things are not really stressful at all. If they don't have stress, they create it.

Even boredom can take a toll. Psychiatrist Dr. Robert Seidenberg has found many women without jobs or absorbing interests suffer a "trauma of eventlessness." Their lives are secure and stable but unfulfilling, because they have no challenge or choices in their lives.

Some people have suggested that personality factors are important to stress. One controversial theory concerning stress-prone men was developed by Drs. Meyer Friedman and Ray Rosenman of San Francisco. They described Type A and B personality patterns. Type A—extremely competitive, striving for achievement, impatient, restless, hyperalert, perfectionist, unable to relax, explosive in speech, with tense face muscles—had twice as many heart attacks as more relaxed Type B men. Type A men had more severe cases and were more likely to develop second attacks.

Now more recent studies show that a hard driving, aggressive, competitive, rushed, job devoted style of life is also associated with a significantly increased risk of coronary heart disease in women.

The experiences of some other researchers suggest that all this may have less to do with inborn personality traits than it has to do with the culture in which these people live and develop. They feel that if people lived in a culture that did not support Type A people, there would be fewer of them.

Evidence that it's not the stressful situation but our reaction to it that is important was found be Dr. Salvatore Maddi of the University of Chicago. He and his associates studied 200 men having highly stressful experiences. Of these, 100 had high illness rates and 100 had low illness rates. The difference? Those who were resistant to illness saw less threat in stress and were much more likely to view changes as an opportunity and a challenge; those who were prone to illness under high stress were more likely to perceive change as a threat.

The cost of our stress culture is high. More Americans die of cardiovascular problems than all other causes of death combined. One out of every three American adults has high blood pressure, and one of the most serious illness costs is associated with hypertension, with its sudden strokes and heart attacks.

The cost is compounded by our reactions to stress. Some of us smoke, drink, overeat, and use tranquilizers and other drugs to help us cope. (The most widely prescribed drug of any kind in the world is one of the tranquilizers.) Others become victims of insomnia, pounding headaches, irritability, indigestion, colitis, sex problems, ulcers, or high blood pressure.

The economic costs are high; some experts put them at $12 billion a year. Others say it is much higher than that. "For executives alone," *The New York Times* reported in November 1978, "one estimate has it that American industry lost between $10 billion and $20 billion annually through lost workdays, hospitalization, and early death caused by stress."

Perhaps the greatest cost of all is that of not being able to live our lives in as enjoyable and relaxed ways as we are capable of.

THE LIFEGAIN PROGRAM FOR MANAGING STRESS

Step One. Understanding Your Own Culture

How many negative norms in your own groups might be contributing to your stress? Check these.

It is a norm in one or more groups that I belong to:

☐ For people to take on more responsibility than they can handle.

☐ For people to worry about their business problems at home and their family problems at work.

☐ For people not to ask for help if their work load becomes too heavy.

☐ For people to work so hard that they tend to lose contact with other important elements of their lives, such as their children, hobbies, recreation.

☐ For people to grow accustomed to and accept the need to live with an almost constant level of stress and tension.

☐ For people to keep feelings bottled up inside rather than express them openly.

☐ For people to move from job to job or city to city—it's the way to get to the top.

☐ For people to work 12 hours a day, seven days a week if they really enjoy their job.

☐ For husbands and wives automatically to argue rather than to approach problems constructively.

☐ For people to wait for problems to disappear instead of facing and dealing with them when they occur.

☐ For people to take out large loans when they're not sure how they can pay them off.

☐ For people to keep on working in a job that does not interest them or does not use their training and abilities.

☐ For people to wait until a supervisor chooses to discuss a problem, rather than to bring it up themselves.

☐ For people to buy things on time when it stretches their budget.

☐ For people not to seek professional help during periods of stress or depression.

☐ For people not to have anyone with whom they can talk over their problems.

How many negative norms did you find? How heavily do they influence you? What would be the effect if all these norms were positive? By reviewing and understanding these norms, you will have taken an important step in understanding how culture affects you and your life in the area of stress control.

Listen for the cues in your life that could mean unwanted stress. Listen for those clicks of the culture traps so you can begin to avoid unnecessary stressful circumstances and begin to build less stressful cultures for yourself.

Step Two. Get The Facts And Separate Fact From Fiction.

You would think with all the talk of stress we would know a lot more about it. But most of us really know very little about stress in general and even less about the stress interactions in our own lives.

TEST YOURSELF ON STRESS FACTS
1. Stress is always negative.   True   False
2. Tranquilizers, alcohol, and sleeping pills have been found very helpful in coping with the everyday pressures of stress.   True   False
3. When a person is suffering from stress, there is little he or she can do to minimize its effects on health.   True   False

4. If you can reduce the number of stress situations you are exposed to in your environment, you can help minimize the physical damage produced by stress in your body.   True   False

5. Stress can adversely affect your sex life.   True   False

6. Everybody has too much stress.   True   False

7. The Type A Coronary Prone Behavior is more common in higher socioeconomic groups and groups with higher education and higher occupational status.   True   False

8. Stress is bad for everybody.   True   False

9. While it is good for you to relax, you need not worry about hypertension until a heart attack or stroke warns you.   True   False

ANSWERS

1. FALSE. "Stress" by itself simply refers to the reaction of the body to a situation. Such a stimulus can be good or bad. It is when the body is repeatedly or constantly into the "fight or flight" stress reaction that damage begins to occur.

2. FALSE. They are useful in crisis situations to reduce anxiety and tension but should not be used on an everyday basis. Better to relieve the underlying problem.

3. FALSE. By using methods of relaxation currently available — TM, biofeedback, the Relaxation Response technique, etc. — you can often reduce your alarm state, with a whole range of physical and mental benefits. You can also minimize the effect by surrounding yourself with people who are learning to deal successfully with stress themselves.

4. TRUE. Obviously, you can reduce the impact of stress on your life by reducing the amount of stress situations you are exposed to, but you must also learn not to overreact to situations. Some people worry before something happens, when it happens, and after it happens, and so are in a chronic state of alarm no matter how few their problems are.

5. TRUE. Prolonged stress can reduce the activity of the sex glands, reduce sexual feeling, and lead to difficulties in sexual activity. This is partly due to the sympathetic nervous system's action and partly due to a shift in hormones given off by the pituitary gland (from making hormones that stimulate the sex glands, to making hormones that counteract stress.)

6. FALSE. Some people suffer from lack of stressors. Bored with routine work or lack of challenge, they may pick fights with their loved ones. Or they may become depressed, gradually accomplishing less and less, or turn to alcoholism, promiscuity, overeating, or gambling. (If you feel understimulated and underinvolved, you may find help in the next chapter with ways to become more involved and to find more excite-

ment and fulfillment in your life.) Some people have overstress in one part of their life and understress in another.

7. TRUE. But only up to a point. Detailed analysis shows that middle managers and professionals have more of the Coronary Prone Behavior Pattern, but the top executives and major professionals who have made it are less likely to be the harried, hurried Type A. And backing up those facts, a 16-year study by Metropolitan Life Insurance of the men who occupy the three top executive positions in the Fortune 500 companies showed them to have a mortality rate that was only 63 percent of that of the rest of the white male population. Perhaps these men had to be more physically and emotionally fit than their contemporaries to get where they were. Perhaps they got to the top because they could handle stress well. Or perhaps the satisfaction of being at the top and being in command is less stressful than making the climb.

8. FALSE. There are two kinds of people in relation to stress, says Dr. Hans Selye, stress expert of the University of Montreal in Canada. And those two kinds of people should set their own pace. "Some people are stress seekers," he says. "They need it to live and be happy. Other people are stress avoiders; they want to be placid and easygoing. Whichever he is, and whatever he does, a person must simply strive to live with his nature and be useful," Selye says. So whether you are a racehorse, a turtle, or something in between, it's necessary for you to contemplate your own personality and what makes you happy. Some people find they have different needs at different times.

9. FALSE. Hypertension, or consistently high blood pressure, can silently build up deposits in the artery walls, hardening them and blocking blood flow without your realizing it. It can cause severe damage to the cardiovascular system or other organs without producing pain or other symptoms. For this reason, it is wise to keep a frequent check on your blood pressure and find ways to decrease it if it is high.

HOW WELL ARE YOU COPING WITH STRESS?

Now check over your management of stress in your own life.

Are you aware of the factors that could be contributing to stress in your life?	Yes	No
Do you regularly check your life for excessive stress and do you know techniques to use to reduce it?	Yes	No
Do you set priorities and schedule your activities to help you avoid feelings of harassment and frustration?	Yes	No
Do you do well in changing stressors in your life?	Yes	No
Do you tell your family and friends if they are producing stress in your life unnecessarily?	Yes	No

Do you keep track of major changes and stress times in your
life and take better care of yourself during clusters of these
stresses to try to avoid the potential negative consequences
of them where possible?   Yes   No

Are you familiar with stress reduction techniques such as
meditation, biofeedback, and deep relaxation?   Yes   No

Do you try to solve problems as soon as possible rather than
hoping that they will go away?   Yes   No

Are you able to avoid being unduly bothered by problems
that you can do little or nothing about at this time?   Yes   No

Do you maintain what you think is for you a successful
balance between work, recreation, and sleep?   Yes   No

Is your work fulfilling and satisfying to you?   Yes   No

Do you sleep well at night and wake most mornings suffi-
ciently rested and ready to start the day?   Yes   No

Are you able to go through the day calmly as opposed to
feeling constantly pressured or harassed?   Yes   No

Do you usually find it easy to relax when there aren't any
tensions in you?   Yes   No

Do you usually find yourself relaxed instead of tuned up
after a short drive or some activity that doesn't require
tension?   Yes   No

Do you find you engage in activities that raise your tension
levels?   Yes   No

Do you regularly find ways to unwind and relax?   Yes   No

Are you able to get away from it all for a least a few minutes
at regular intervals?   Yes   No

Are you able to keep minor problems and disappointments
from upsetting you?   Yes   No

Do you spend 10 to 20 minutes a day on relaxation?   Yes   No

If you answered *yes* to all questions, you are probably handling stress very
well in your life.

If you had some *no* responses, you can probably learn a great deal in this
chapter on better ways to manage stress to help you have a more satisfying
and enjoyable life.

Clues From Your Hidden Tensions.   Here are tension clues to look for. You
might even have some of them right now.

☐   Butterflies in the stomach

☐   Eyes fluttering or eyestrain

☐   Tight neck or jaw muscles

☐   Chin jutted out, biting or grinding teeth

☐   Sweating palms, feet, or armpits

- ☐ Cold hands
- ☐ General irritability or depression
- ☐ High pulse rate
- ☐ Moving too brusquely, muscles tight or braced
- ☐ Irregular shallow breathing or sighing respiration
- ☐ Tight strained voice
- ☐ Shoulders hunched
- ☐ Toes or fingers tightly curled
- ☐ Spine rigid
- ☐ Forehead tight, sometimes with a headache beginning
- ☐ Heart pounding
- ☐ Unusually dry throat or mouth
- ☐ Strong urge to run, hide, or cry out
- ☐ Lack of concentration
- ☐ General fatigue
- ☐ Persistently keyed up
- ☐ Easily startled
- ☐ Can't sit still
- ☐ Grinding of teeth
- ☐ Change in appetite
- ☐ Nightmares

WHEN CHANGES TAKE PLACE TOO FAST — A LIFE CHANGE TEST TO ANALYZE STRESS

Drs. Thomas Holmes and Richard Rahe, psychiatrists at the University of Washington in Seattle, have devised a scale to help predict illness that comes from too much stress. They find that any change, good or bad, can produce stress, and that major illness often follows when a person has many stress-related changes that occur in one year. If a stress is severe enough, they found, it may be related to whether you develop a disease, when you develop it, and how severe it is.

The following Life Change Index lists the life events that appear to affect health with the point value the scientists assigned for them. While times have changed so point values might be different, you might still like to read the list of stressful circumstances, check the ones that have occurred to you in the past 12 months, and total your score to have an indication of how much stress you have experienced. You can also use the test to estimate how much stress you will be under from events you know are about to happen in the near future.

LIFE CHANGE INDEX

Event	Scale of Impact
Death of Spouse	100
Divorce	73
Marital Separation	65
Jail Term	63
Death of Close Family Member	63
Personal Injury or Illness	53
Marriage	50
Fired at Work	47
Marital Reconciliation	45
Retirement	45
Change in Health of Family Member	44
Pregnancy	40
Sex Difficulties	39
Gain of New Family Member	39
Business Readjustment	39
Change in Financial State	38
Death of a Close Friend	37
Change to Different Line of Work	36
Change in Number of Arguments with Spouse	35
Mortgage over $10,000	31
Foreclosure of Mortgage or Loan	30
Change in Responsibilities at Work	29
Son or Daughter Leaving Home	29
Trouble with In-Laws	29
Outstanding Personal Achievement	28
Spouse Begins or Stops Work	26
Begin or End School	26
Change in Living Conditions	25
Revision of Personal Habits	24
Trouble with Boss	23
Change in Work Hours or Conditions	20
Change in Residence	20
Change in Schools	20
Change in Recreation	19
Change in Church Activities	19
Change in Social Activities	18
Mortgage or Loan Less Than $10,000	17
Change in Sleeping Habits	16
Change in Number of Family Get-Togethers	15
Change in Eating Habits	15
Vacation	13
Christmas (if approaching)	12
Minor Violation of the Law	11

In the persons studied, 79 percent became severely ill within a year if the changes occurring in life totaled over 300 points. You may feel that some of these events might have a different stress score than those given and may want to make some adjustments.

If your score is beyond the dangerous 300 mark, you should seriously consider some changes to make your life less stressful and to obtain professional assistance if necessary.

Step Three. Find Or Build Yourself A Supportive Environment

Many times the people who surround us contribute to our stress problem rather than alleviate it without our or their being aware of it.

Picture Jim Holcombe. He works almost twice as many hours as he should be doing. His boss appreciates him for the hard worker he is. "It would take two to replace him." His wife appreciates it because he earns a good living. She just can't understand why he can't be home more often to help around the house. His co-workers appreciate it; Jim can really be relied upon. He'll do his part and more. Even his parents are proud of him. "He's a hard worker. If only he would take the time to visit us more often." Jim's high school extols him. He was invited back to speak at graduation and introduced as the one in his class voted "most likely to succeed"—and he did. His college invites him back every year to participate in career day. His church board recently elected him president, saying, "If you want something done, you ask the busiest man."

Mary Jane is similarly influenced by people who praise her for being a superwoman. She cooks great meals and is always there to help if there is a problem. Her husband and children find her a little tense though, and they can't understand why she doesn't relax a bit.

And so it goes. We surround ourselves with people who support our bad health practices, including those who add stress to our already stressful lives. Somehow we have to alter these patterns in our lives. It may be helpful to have a husband or wife, or even a whole family participate in the Lifegain program at the same time.

Where the people who surround us can't or won't change, it may be necessary for us to find new support groups. Perhaps Jim Holcombe's friends will have less vested interest in his being such a hard worker and superachiever than his family and co-workers do. Maybe the women's consciousness raising group that Mary Jane goes to will not provide her with quite the same level of encouragement for "killing herself" and making sure she does everything just "right" as her family does.

Your Lifegain support group should be helpful to you in supporting your efforts at change. You may also want to get some special instruction in relaxation techniques. They are available in many locations. Try your universities, local Y's, or health clubs.

Check your doctor, a psychologist, a psychiatrist, a local clinic, or even the telephone book for instruction in biofeedback. TM, yoga, time management, and other techniques for reducing stress are sometimes taught in clinics. Some cities even have special stress reduction centers, using one or more of these relaxation techniques. Sometimes workshops are sponsored by local Y's or health clubs. Some companies are now offering stress reduction workshops for their employees. Some even provide quiet rooms and have reported good results with them.

And, as with any of the Lifegain programs, you can set up your own groups to meet weekly or monthly to bring materials together, tell experiences, and give each other support.

Check your library and local bookstore for some of the many good books and tapes on stress, management of time, and relaxation techniques.

MAKING THE DECISION

You've read the facts and you've analyzed how much stress there is in your life. If you think you have too much hidden stress, if you feel you're not coping with stress as well as you'd like, decide what you would like to do about it.

To get a feeling of where you are at this point, indicate below how many of the following commitments you are personally prepared to make.

☐ I am prepared to help change some aspect of the wider environment that seems to me to be particularly stressful in a negative way, such as:

_____

_____

☐ I am prepared to change some particularly stressful aspect of my personal environment, such as:

_____

_____

☐ I feel there are some stressful aspects of my environment I cannot change and will have to accept. They are:

_____

_____

☐ I am devoting at least one-half hour a day (preferably in two separate periods) to complete personal relaxation through a technique such as the Relaxation Response or meditation.

If you want to learn to manage stress better, read through the suggestions and illustrations that follow and decide which ones to put into action yourself.

And even before you start your action plan, begin to picture yourself as a relaxed person at work, at home, and socially. Begin to feel what it's like when you are stressed and when you are relaxed.

When you make your commitment to change, tell someone about it. Having others know your plans will motivate you further to carry them out.

Step Four. Some Ideas That Might Help

While we probably can't eliminate all stressful situations from our lives (and perhaps we wouldn't even want to), we can eliminate some stress input and reduce the harmful aspect of what remains with specific workable techniques. President Kennedy used to lean back on the wall, close his eyes, and completely relax whenever free moments came, even in elevators. Henry Ford said he could handle difficult jobs by breaking them down to small components and working on each in turn. Dr. Paul Dudley White rode his bike and walked for miles. Several famous people use slow deep breathing and progressive relaxation exercises. One network science editor hums before going on the air. A famous surgeon sighs before he cuts. President Eisenhower, when feeling stress before a speech, would picture everyone in the front row wearing underwear.

In the following pages we give you a variety of techniques, some to reduce stress situations and some to cope with stress as it occurs. Pick one or two that you think will be most effective for you. Practice it every day, tracking your progress. If it doesn't work, switch to another method. We have purposely included many techniques, so you can find the one best for you.

YOU CAN REDUCE STRESS BY CHANGING HOW YOU SEE THINGS

As one workshop participant said, "I finally learned there is nothing to be gained by working myself up. I simply don't let my insides get as involved as I used to."

The key is to learn relaxed thinking. In the final analysis, it isn't the stressful situation itself that usually causes the problem; it's our attitude toward the situation, our reaction to it. It's how we perceive the situation.

A burned dinner, milk spilled, a flat tire, a bill unpaid, a job lost, a child crying; all are potentially stressful situations. But how much they affect us and our health depends on the way we react to them. We don't need to have a frenzied, rushed, tense, seething, aggressive, anxious, tense reaction to life. We can learn to do otherwise.

YOU CAN REDUCE STRESS BY WATCHING FOR HIDDEN TENSION EVERY DAY

Everybody has tension occasionally when things go wrong, but some people are tense almost constantly without knowing it.

Check yourself periodically when you are working or solving problems to see whether you have a relaxed use of energy or are uptight and hurrying for no good reason.

When you feel signs of tension coming on, take deep breaths and take a minute to relax. Let your muscles go limp, then resume your activity but slow your pace.

YOU CAN REDUCE STRESS BY ORGANIZING YOUR LIFE

If your life is full of conflicting demands, rushing here and there, never seeming to get anything done, then simplify and organize.

Think about how you spend your days. Eliminate all the unnecessary tasks you can, and identify needed and desired activities, so you are not always in a frenzy struggling against time.

Keep lists: one for shopping and one for what you want to do (include recreational things). Underline priority items so you will get these done for sure. Be a perfectionist on important things but not on low priority things.

Learn to concentrate on a task when you do it. Don't let your mind wander to other problems while you're doing this one.

Use small bits of time. Watch only the television programs really important to you. Use an hour in the evening for a family hobby or to get a small job done. Carry a book to read, letters to write, or other small projects with you, so you can take advantage of any waiting or commuting time.

To help make time for the jobs and pleasures you really want, get help for less important jobs you can afford to delegate.

Then — and this is vital — learn how to say *no* to things you don't really want to do.

And finally — take time to relax. Set aside time for it, and make sure it's relaxing for you. What is relaxing for one person is not necessarily relaxing for another. Read through the techniques below and see what suits you.

YOU CAN REDUCE STRESS WITH MEDITATION
AND OTHER RELAXATION TECHNIQUES

Some people find that an effective way to break the stress cycle is by regularly practicing deep muscle relaxation or meditation. If you choose to use one of these techniques, you will find it much easier to keep up if you make it a regular built-in part of your life, setting aside a specific time each day, such as before lunch or dinner. To experience meditation, find a quiet place, sit in a comfortable position, and close your eyes. Take a deep, slow, long breath. Let calmness come into your body. Let your muscles relax, your mind blank to nothing, drifting. Just let it happen. Observe it, the feeling of peace and serenity, but don't try to control it.

There are many varieties of meditation techniques. With some you let your mind wander as it wishes; in some techniques, such as TM, you keep saying one word or phrase over and over to keep your mind from wandering.

In Yoga or Zen meditation you center on respiration; in some you practice an exercise called one-pointing in which you contemplate a pleasant object, focusing your gaze on a lighted candle, a leaf, a flower, or on still water, feeling and appreciating its form and detail. Tai Chi combines movement with meditation, giving you the added advantage of exercise while you concentrate.

People who practice sitting meditation generally use the technique for 10 to 20 minutes twice a day but not within two hours after any meal. Done regularly, it frequently has been shown to reduce tension and anxiety, lower blood pressure, decrease occurrences of irregular heartbeats, and help smokers, drug users, and alcoholics quit.

Progressive Relaxation. Remove or loosen any tight clothing. Lie on your back, close your eyes. Breathe in deeply (through the nose) and raise your arms over your head. Hold your breath and stretch, tensing all muscles, then let them go limp and exhale slowly (through the nose), dropping your arms to your side. Now lie limply, and take another long, deep breath. Exhale as far as you can, releasing your breath very slowly.

Starting with your feet, tense your muscles then let go. First the toes of your right foot. Tense; relax; then the toes of your left foot. Now gradually tense and relax the ankles, calves, knees, and thighs until your legs feel loose and free. Let waves of relaxation spread into your abdomen, chest, and shoulders; then all along your spine and back. Feel the muscles begin to loosen. Tense your abdominal muscles; relax. Tighten your buttocks and relax. Now relax your fingers one by one. Close and open your fists, first your right hand, then your left. Relax the muscles in your arm. Shrug your shoulders, then relax. Relax along the sides and back of your neck. Tense your facial muscles, then relax. Let your jaw sag with lips slightly parted. Yawn. Feel your scalp loosen. Let your eyes relax and rest. Feel the relaxation enveloping your entire body. Become aware of the steady, slow beating of your heart and of your breath as it flows in and out. Breathe in deeply, breathing in energy from around you. As you breathe out, more and more tension leaves you. Concentrate on the flow of your breath and feel the state of relaxed peace.

The Rag Doll. Stand with your legs apart and bend at the waist. Let your head and arms hang. Shake your arms and hands loosely. Sway from side to side.

Imagery. Lie down and imagine a series of numbers being painted slowly in the sky, or picture yourself drifting lazily on a cloud, or floating softly on a warm balmy Bahamian sea. Or as you lie on your back completely relaxed, imagine you are a sponge, limp, loose, and inert. Press your neck and back into the sofa, bed, or floor. Close your eyes, breathe deeply through your nose, relax each part of your body, and let your body, like a sponge, soak up strength and tranquility.

Abdominal Breathing. Lie flat on your back, place one hand on your abdomen and one on your chest, so you can feel that you are breathing with the abdomen, not the chest. Inhale deeply and slowly through the nostrils and expand the abdomen without pulling the air up to the chest. Keep your shoulders and chest relaxed. Exhale slowly through the nostrils while pulling the abdomen to the back of the spine. Some people like to do abdominal breathing with feet elevated and head down on a slant board.

The Sighing Breath. Inhale deeply through the nostrils to the count of eight, then with lips puckered (as if cooling soup) exhale very slowly through the mouth to the count of 16 or as long as you can. Concentrate on the long sighing sound and feel the tension dissolve. Repeat at least 10 times. One man who complained of tension headaches for 20 years cut his tension by breathing exercises, and his headaches disappeared in just three weeks.

The Neck-Relaxers Head Bounce. Tilt your left ear to your left shoulder several times in a bouncing motion. Then bounce the right ear to the right shoulder several times. Then do a head roll, circling your head around loosely in one direction, then the other. Or to use a chiropractor-osteopath technique, curl your fingers around the side of your neck, meeting in back. Lift up and forward as though you were trying to lift your head off your shoulders. Turn your head slightly from right to left while you continue lifting.

Do-It-Yourself Head And Neck Massage. Close your eyes and massage your head and neck in firm small circles. With your head and neck limp, massage the skull, then massage down along the neck vertebrae to the shoulders.

Common Sense Remedies. A good hot tub or shower, a hot cup of tea, a nap, getting up frequently and stretching after you have been sitting at a desk or on a trip for a long time.

BIOFEEDBACK

With biofeedback you learn to control the autonomic functions of your body by monitoring body functions on a machine that uses meters, sounds, or flashing lights to tell you the effect you are producing on muscle tension, skin temperature, heart rate, blood pressure, or other functions. You sit there with electrodes attached to your forehead and hands and simply imagine the change you want. The machine in front of you shows any changes produced, tells you whether you're tense or relaxed. The biofeed-back technique has also proved helpful in treating headaches, high blood pressure, ulcers, Raynaud's disease, insomnia, phobias, anxiety states, asthma, epilepsy, heart arrhythmias, and speech problems. Some biofeedback laboratories, such as the Stress Transformation Center in New York, are open to the public; for some centers, persons must be referred by a psychologist or physician.

OTHER WAYS TO RELIEVE STRESS

Try to calm your sense of time urgency. You don't have to rush through the day as if you're running in a race. Nobody is holding a stop watch on you. Take a deep breath and walk a little slower.

Ask yourself a question. Is this matter going to be important five minutes from now? If not, maybe it's not worth getting upset about, especially if you can't do anything about it.

Escape for a while. Go to a movie, visit a friend, play a game with your child. But make it only a short escape, then come back and deal with your difficulty.

Learn to live day by day, moment by moment, and find some enjoyment and beauty in each day. Try the Buddha philosophy of paying attention to the here and now, savoring eating when you're eating, or concentrating only on driving when you are driving and not on something else in the past or future.

Please yourself. You deserve a break today and every day. Pamper yourself. Have a massage, take a leisurely walk, buy yourself a present, have a manicure, do nothing, sleep late without feeling guilty. Do something just for the fun of it.

Try to find work you really like. It isn't the stress of work that wears us out but the stress of frustration and failure. Working long hours, doing hard physical labor, or commuting several hours a day to work, rarely lead to the types of stress symptoms which endanger a person's health or ability to function. One study of 800 executives over a three-year period showed no correlation between anxiety level and items like salary, number of hours worked, or number of hours spent commuting. But there was a correlation between anxiety and whether or not there was satisfaction with a job.

Use music as therapy. Listening to a tranquil classic helps sooth nerves in curb to curb traffic. Losing yourself to the rhythm of dancing can help you let off steam. Listening to the beat of blues or jazz can ease the tensions from your soul.

When you relax, really relax. Some people watch TV and still are tense, lie on a beach and worry about the office. Put your problems out of your mind and lose yourself to relaxing.

Consider religion or read the philosophers. It gives many people a sense of purpose and peace that helps put oil on the waters of stress situations.

Call a friend. It helps to lean on someone in time of crisis. Let a friend know you really need help. If that isn't enough, consider professional help.

Enjoy your family. Whether it's with your parents, your spouse, or your children, you can help relax your stress overload with understanding and support as well as enjoyment together.

Don't worry so much about money. Most men would rather have a loving understanding wife than a bigger house. Most women prefer a husband's tenderness and attention to a fur coat. Most kids wouldn't mind making do with a simple second-hand bike instead of a new 10 speed if they had plenty of love and attention and some time with their parents.

Try creative daydreaming. If you have a problem, try to imagine various solutions to it and what their consequences would be. This changes non-productive worry into energy used for a solution.

Assess your skills at your job. If you are tense because you feel inadequate at your job, take some courses or read books to improve your skills or try to switch to another job you think will fit you better.

Talk to your employer. Two of the biggest causes of stress on the job are not having clear work objectives, so you know what is expected, and not having adequate facts or tools to do a job. Both could be solved by non-hostile discussions with your boss.

Try cooperation instead of competition. You don't always have to edge out the other person on the highway or win a discussion. Stop being a threat to others and they may stop being a threat to you.

Don't try to be a superperson. You can't be perfect. Give the best of your efforts and ability, but don't feel guilty if you don't achieve the impossible.

Consider changing your diet. Your diet can affect whether you tend to be tense or tranquil. Try reducing the caffeine in your diet and eliminating medicines with caffeine, such as headache pills. Try eliminating sugar from your diet, completely avoiding table sugar and all foods and drinks that contain sugar. If you have wide fluctuations in sugar levels in your blood, try smoothing them out by eating a snack of cheese, nuts, eggs, or meat every three hours.

Do something physical. If you feel pent-up anger or frustration, cool off by gardening or cleaning out the garage. Take a walk, jog, skip rope, run, play tennis, golf, go to a dance, climb, swim. Do anything to start working it out.

Exercise. Regular exercise has been shown to reduce stress and the effects of stress greatly. Put on your schedule a half hour of walking a day for at least three days a week, and a half hour of light calisthenics at least three days a week. You can alternate these, one day a walk, the next day calisthenics, etc. And increase your activities along with it, walking up that extra flight of stairs, washing the car, taking a swim.

In addition to helping relieve stress, this extra exercise will also improve your cardiovascular functioning and bring you other benefits.

Step Five. Keep Track And Tune In

It's so easy for stress to creep back into our lifestyles that it's necessary to check regularly for hidden tensions.

One family in Detroit kept track of their progress by setting up two tables — one for how they rated their stress level (Table 1), and the other for how beneficial they thought their stress control exercises were that

TABLE 1. Daily Stress Levels

	VERY RELAXED	RATHER RELAXED	RATHER TENSE	VERY TENSE
Mon.				
Tues.				
Wed.				
Thur.				
Fri.				
Sat.				
Sun.				

day (Table 2). They set aside a few minutes each evening to think about and record on a list their experiences that day.

Sherry Salem is a high-powered public relations consultant who runs press rooms for national meetings with phones jingling, cameramen yelling, and 10 reporters at once all wanting interviews so they can make their deadlines. There was no way to eliminate stress from her job, but she learned to apply coping techniques, and now keeps track of her tension by simply pausing several times during the hectic times and mentally checking herself for tight muscles, shaking, pounding when she walks. "The very act of checking helps keep you from being unnecessarily tense," she says. "And each day that I

TABLE 2. Relaxation Training Effectiveness

	VERY	SOMEWHAT	NOT AT ALL
Mon.			
Tues.			
Wed.			
Thur.			
Fri.			
Sat.			
Sun.			

use the check-it-out-and-cool-it techniques I find I have progressed a little more to being less tense."

Helen M., who used to scrub floors grimly, pound up and down the steps to do the laundry, and wash dishes with muscles so tense she could have snapped each plate in two, found that the same periodic checking helped her. She used the hidden tension test on page 174 whenever she thought of it as she did the housework, and was impressed with how much progress she was making toward less tension.

As you first work to manage your stress, check frequently, reinforcing your own good actions, helping to set up the new good habits. When not being tense has become a normal thing, you can check your reactions less frequently, only doing so occasionally or at special crisis times.

Step Six. Reward Yourself And Have Fun

When you're in love your step is bouncy, your grin is wide, and the world sparkles back at you. We don't guarantee you all of that if you learn to cope with stress, but you will feel a weight lift from your shoulders, the tightness leave you, and a sense of tranquility replace some of the frustration and tension that was raging through your body.

When you get that sense of being right with the world, your attitude changes and you become relaxed enough to automatically be programmed for fun.

Bonnie Gonzalez of New York City had been married for two years and found she was constantly bickering with her husband. Everything was criticism or a fight between them. Tension and irritability seemed to be the way of operating with her parents and with her friends too. Bonnie started on the Lifegain stress program and found she could control her tensions better. But every time she got back with her old friends and the people at her job, the old pattern would come back.

"I just couldn't make the change stick," she said. "And I couldn't go on operating the way I was. I could change myself on a temporary basis, but pretty soon the outbursts of temper and the tension of my family and job and my old gang soon had me back in the same old mold." But with support from her new Lifegain workshop friends, she began discussing the tension situations with her family and friends.

"It made all the difference in the world. Once you have become involved with others, then you can help each other. Pretty soon it got to the point when someone exploded, we'd say 'Be careful, your stress is showing.' It got to be a group joke, and with time we actually saw our patterns of behavior changing. Being more calm and relaxed was supported by everyone and became a part of our daily living.

"Then we built in some rewards for ourselves both individually and as a group. I bought myself some good hiking shoes because I found I liked relaxing best in the woods, and as a group we rewarded ourselves by going to comedy plays and movies together whenever they came to the neighborhood.

"I'm a different person now. I have an absolute ball."

Step Seven. Reach Out To Others

As birth is the first place we experience stress, so it may be the first place we can help ease stress for others.

Many obstetricians are finding good results with the method of Dr. F. Leboyer (Birth Without Violence) in which the baby is laid on its mother's abdomen at delivery, softly touched, and allowed to begin breathing naturally while the umbilical cord is left attached until all its blood has reached the baby. Then the newborn is gently washed in a warm water bath and cradled in its mother's arms. Throughout infancy Dr. Leboyer encourages parents to touch their infants, to caress them, massage them, rock them.

Many mothers are adopting the soothing technique of mothers in India who use a touch massage on their infants to reduce stress. They use an oil for the massage; sensitively, lightly, gently, responsively speaking to the baby with their hands, following the body contours slowly, soothingly, and lovingly; then they support the baby in warm bath water for a few moments more of total relaxation.

Older children can be helped to deal with stress, too. Be sensitive to their problems, listen, be understanding, help them be as free as possible of worry and tension, and help them learn to cope with tension when it's necessary. Children can be taught to solve problems with a minimum of stress reaction. Solving problems creatively and calmly is a matter of practice and of seeing other people act that way. You can also help to prepare them for stress situations by explaining things to them in advance. Talk with them about the first day of school, the first trip to the dentist, and what it will be like.

As your children get older, explore with them the pressures they will be facing in high school: peer pressures on smoking, drinking, driving, pot. Let them know that you understand those pressures, and talk about ways they can make decisions that are best for themselves.

But probably the simplest way to reduce stress for your children is to make every effort possible to eliminate bickering and put-downs and encourage a peaceful and cooperative family life. Enjoy each other!

You can reach out to adults too. Talk to people where you work about ways stress could be reduced. Have people describe what they consider stressful about their work and see if changes can be made.

Understand your spouse's stresses, whether it's housewife syndrome or fear of being fired from a job, and do what you can to alleviate the other's tensions.

Try not to be a stress carrier. Marvin, an executive in a large manufacturing firm, found he was such a carrier. "I used to keep people guessing about where they stood," he says. "I would try to put people under heavy pressure all the time, thinking they'd work better. I would lay my problems on other people and then get angry when they tried to help. And I would bring my tensions home without explaining the reason so people could understand." Now Marvin has changed. If he sees someone who is already harassed, he tries not to add to their problems. He's more relaxed, and so are the people who work with him.

One of the keys to stress seems to be that so often we are facing our problems alone, battling our day-to-day crises without help or encouragement. So one of the biggest helps we can give the person under stress is our emotional support. Do whatever you can to increase your efforts at assistance and support, even to such simple things as helping with shopping, shoveling snow, or other chores. Get other people to be supportive also if you can; and if it's necessary, get the person to a doctor or psychologist for professional support. You probably know at least one person right now having difficulty in a marriage, at work, or at school. Let them know you care.

12

How To Get Along With Yourself and Others

A very clever cartoon showed two dolphins cavorting through the water with one saying to the other: "Although humans make sounds with their mouths and occasionally look at each other, there is no solid evidence that they actually communicate among themselves."*

We live in a culture that frequently robs us of the enjoyment of our own lives and of the lives of those around us.

And moreover this happens without our really being aware of what has happened to us.

For too many of us life becomes a struggle to be survived rather than a joy to be celebrated. We treat ourselves to indignities and put-downs that we would be shocked to hear from others. Most of us would be up in arms if others called us lazy or stupid, but we feel free to accept that kind of appellation from ourselves.

Most of us would tell a boss to drop dead if he required us to worry about our jobs all of our working hours and weekends, too; and we sometimes make those kinds of demands upon ourselves.

Unfortunately it is the norm in our culture to accept and even expect this kind of treatment for ourselves. After all, we say, if I can't be honest with myself how am I going to know the truth about myself? But is this the truth, or is it merely a culturally supported distortion that interferes with our being the kind of people that we are capable of being?

Psychoanalyst Karen Horney presented a very valuable tool for analyzing this characteristic phenomenon within ourselves. She talked about it as the "idealized self-image." When you are born, she explains, you have an actual self, and that actual self is a dynamic moving characteristic. It's all you are now plus all you're capable of becoming. What happens is that the society tells you that your actual self is not adequate. (This often happens to the child who is learning to eat, when the small muscle control is not sufficient to allow him to get the spoon to the mouth. When he fails and gets food on himself, the mother says, "How could you do that?" or "If you were as good as you should be you wouldn't do that!" The same sequence also often occurs during toilet training, when the child is asked to control his sphincter and bowel movement before he is physically able to accomplish it.)

So we create in our minds an image of the type of person we need to be to

*Sidney Harris, *What's So Funny About Science?* Los Altos, Ca.: American Scientist, 1977.

be fully acceptable, and then we reach for the image. When we don't achieve it, which by definition we can't, we come back to the only place possible — the actual self. We wipe that out as an acceptable alternative and come down through it, finally, to create a new image, the image of our despised self — the self that is not good enough to be fully accepted either by ourselves or others.

Unfortunately, we often extend this same negative approach to our relationships with others, pointing out the few flaws we see in their behavior rather than the many strengths. We extol the virtues of our separateness and independence when our relatedness and our interdependence are actually what makes us most uniquely human. We often forget that humans are by their inheritance social beings and require a long period of interrelationships in order to survive. The human infant would almost certainly die within less than five years if social relationships with others of its species were not available.

Our relationships with others are frequently distant and isolated. Our living arrangements contribute to this isolation. We were recently told of an aborigine group from central Australia who were invited to a conference in a motel setting in one of Australia's modern cities. Each of the 15 participants was assigned a separate room in the motel. Not understanding why this should be and not wanting to be isolated and separated from one another, the group moved into a single room, leaving the other 14 rooms vacant. The organizers of the conference were amazed at this and perhaps did not recognize the high price that all of us pay for the isolation that we are pushing upon ourselves.

While overcrowding is probably not the answer to loneliness and isolation, it is clear that from a mental health standpoint there are a number of problems resulting from the separateness of our lives. Ashley Montagu, one of our leading contemporary anthropologists, has drawn attention to the tragic failure of our culture to encourage people to be in close physical contact with one another. In his book, *Touching*, he points out that touching occurs in every mammal ever studied, and in fact, newborn animals do not begin to function completely until licked, nuzzled, and fondled. Newborn lambs, not licked, will not stand and will subsequently die. And conversely, animals regularly handled by laboratory workers are found to grow faster, learn better, be gentler, cope better with stress, and live longer. Even premature infants have become healthier and more active and grown faster when regularly stroked every day in addition to being given the usual nursery care.

We need to put mothers and newborn infants in the hospital together again. We need to bring back rocking chairs and mothers and fathers, too, who will rock their children, hug them, and carry them about. We need touching by both men and women. How few men know how to touch women gently and lovingly, how to handle children gently. How rare it is for a father to put his arms around his son. And the untouched son grows up to be the untouched man who in turn does not touch his son.

It would not be quite so bad if these things were happening to us through our free and open choice, but for the most part they are not. They are being foisted upon us by a culture that causes many people to feel that there are no alternatives and that it's a matter of human nature rather than cultural choice that is causing our difficulties.

If we choose to live in isolated, stress-torn, competitive, alienated cultures, that's our business, but to have this foisted upon us as the only alternative is another story entirely.

And our professional approach is not helping either.

We live in a culture that emphasizes the avoidance of mental illness instead of obtaining optimal mental health. As in other health areas, our attention is almost exclusively on correcting problems that have already occurred instead of on increasing potentials within us.

Mental health experts have spent nearly all of their time studying a small percentage of the population for their individual pathology and almost none of their time looking at the characteristics of good mental health, learning how people can bring the most joy and happiness and satisfaction to their lives to reach their highest potential of self-actualization.

Too often mental health has been defined as the absence of mental illness. But just because we're not mentally ill doesn't mean we're mentally healthy. Lifegain defines mental health as living up to our full potential as human beings in our relationship with ourselves and with others and with our universe, having the ability to fully enjoy life and to contribute to the enjoyment of life by others.

Using that definition of mental health, our culture turns out to be not very supportive, with its admonitions and put-downs, frequent pomposities, and our holding in of our feelings. In fact, the culture surrounding us frequently contributes less to our fun and to our self-realization than it does to our anxiety and our unhappiness.

In mental health more than in any other area, our culture puts ceilings on our minds. It expects us to adjust to norms which we might not choose for ourselves. It lays out narrow expected paths to choose, like products in a department store but it does not encourage us either to ask whether there are any other paths or to make our own.

We learn to adjust.

But the norms we are expected to adjust to often prevent us from being what we want to be and block us from reaching our potential with ourselves and others. And the emphasis on adjustment itself is another negative characteristic of many of our cultures.

"Be yourself," some would say. "It's all up to you." But social norms which oppose us cause confusion and conflict and often sabotage our attempts to do what we really want to do.

We yearn for a chance to be appreciated. We'd like someone to listen to our ideas at home and on the job. We'd like to make more friends, good friends. We would like to find more love and understanding in our lives, more satisfaction in our day-to-day living.

But our cultures do not support self-actualization. They trap us on narrow paths. They get in the way of our creativity and imagination, squelch feelings, prevent achievement, foster guilt, discourage personal pleasures, inhibit curiosity and adventure, demand conformity, require obedience to dull and routine work.

Our families often put down the child who is different or discourage the person who wants to try a unique career.

In schools, rigid schedules usually determine what subjects students may study, what interests they have time to follow. Interests, sometimes entire careers, are often in response to fads manufactured by business, or popular events, or trends that determine money available for scholarships and research grants.

Businesses typecast people, and despite antidiscrimination laws, turn down people for jobs or promotions if they do not conform. Norms often dictate the stages of career development, and some, like retirement, are written into legal presentations.

Our economic system buys us leisure, but our culture encourages us not to use it fully. Television viewing replaces conversation among family and friends. The discussions we do have are often unimaginative, carefully skirting controversial or deep discussions of topics important to us. Our culture has encouraged us to forget how to share, to listen, to communicate. Men are not encouraged to show tenderness.

We're discouraged from reaching out to others in meaningful ways or to ask for help.

For many of us, our relationships are less than we would want them to be. We stand at the graves of our relatives and friends and wonder why we weren't able to talk more and show more. We struggle through our days, growing with an emptiness, feeling that we are not quite able to grasp happiness. We reach old age wondering where our dreams went.

What do we want for ourselves?

Is it only to fight our way to money and status, a bigger house and swimming pool? Is it only to fight tensions and anxieties all our lives, so we can sit in a rocking chair when we're older, or go to a nursing home and vegetate, or be at the end of a plastic tube in a hospital? We know there must be more to fulfillment than this, but often we feel that we're not finding that something more.

Our not attaining our potential in mental health, just like our not reaching our potential in physical health, costs us dearly both personally and economically.

We spend nearly $3 billion a year — half a million dollars a day — on mental illness services. Emotional problems cost business and our economy $20 billion a year in lost productive time.

With all these expenditures, we are doing little either to contribute to mental health or to care for those who are mentally ill. Our lack of caring communities, our mental hospitals, and mental illness systems often create as many problems as they manage to cure. Our noncaring communities often treat people with disdain when they return from periods of hospitalization.

The tragedy of this is even more clear when we realize that more than six million people receive treatment in mental institutions, through outpatient clinics, and on psychiatrists' couches. And the President's Commission on Mental Health recently reported that up to 32 million of us may actually be in need of professional help.

Some experts estimate that one in ten of us will at one time in our lives suffer mental or emotional illnesses that will require professional help.

Physicians estimate that as many as half of all medical and surgical problems they treat are rooted in emotional problems.

But perhaps the greatest cost is in our lost lives. Unfortunately, most of us are living out our lives without reaching our full potential, without finding the path right for ourselves, without finding satisfaction with ourselves and with others.

Fortunately, it doesn't need to be that way, and there are a number of things that we can do about it. Some of these may already be beginning to occur.

THE LIFEGAIN MENTAL HEALTH PROGRAM

Step One. Understanding Your Own Culture

Probably more than any other health practice, mental health habits are influenced by the culture around you. So to understand how you relate to that cultural base your first step is to lift the ceiling off your mind.

Culture puts a lid on our thinking, keeping us from believing we can change, from understanding what kind of obstacles we face, from seeing the way we can work together to bring about change.

Cultural factors impinge on a person's attitudes, values, and behavior every day. But as in all Lifegain programs you can use your knowledge of cultural influences to your advantage. If you are not reaching your full potential, and few of us are, understanding the cultural basis for your problems can give you power to confront negative norms and grab on to the things you know are better.

Instead of viewing emotional problems as a strictly individual matter, you can begin to look at them as the outgrowth of a culture that promotes negative mental health norms.

Initially it is difficult, but gradually we can begin to realize that we have been automatically responding to many subgroups — our family, job, friends, social groups, neighbors — and have actually learned to behave in accordance with their expectations rather than carving out our own criteria. Few people realize the far-reaching impact a culture has on our mental and emotional development, things that we consider "human nature."

Evaluating how our cultural experiences have influenced our behavior constitutes the first step in your Lifegain program.

Check the attitudes and behaviors in your various groups. Is it a norm in your groups:

☐ for many people not to live up to the potential that they possess?

☐ for people not to get as much out of life as they are capable of getting?

☐ for many people to be inflexible and uptight in their lifestyle?

☐ for people to cut themselves off from others?

☐ for people not to have sufficient enjoyment in their lives?

☐ for people not to be able to take risks, to experiment, to add a sense of freedom and adventure to their lives?

☐ for people to put unnecessary obstacles in the way of their own achievement?

☐ for people not to work together as well as they could?

☐ for people to hold back on expressing positive feelings, saying positive things to others?

☐ for people to be less effective in their human relations skills than they might be?

☐ for people to think it's unmanly to show love and tenderness?

☐ for people to think it's sissy to enjoy art and good books?

☐ for people to consider it normal for families to bicker and yell?

☐ for people to say "after the kids are gone then we'll. . ."?

☐ for people to think you should keep your problems to yourself; no one else wants to hear them?

☐ for people to feel it's silly to bother your doctor with emotional problems; he's there for your physical health?

☐ for people to be embarrassed to see a psychiatrist or professional counselor?

☐ for people to hide any emotional problems, figuring others will think they're odd?

☐ for people to routinely put up with situations that are disturbing, frustrating, anxiety-producing?

☐ for people to feel it's normal to be depressed; everybody feels down a lot, that it's a crummy world?

☐ for people to be afraid to talk to strangers because they might be rejected or misunderstood?

☐ for people to hold back, afraid to touch people physically or emotionally?

☐ for people to hold in hurts, angers, and problems instead of trying to work them out?

☐ for people to feel isolated from one another?

By understanding the common attitudes in the cultural groups that surround us, we can begin to analyze how we came by some of our beliefs and practices. Then we can choose which ones we really want to keep and which ones we would prefer to change.

Changing just a few of these practices can remarkably change your life.

Step Two. Get The Facts And Separate Fact From Fiction

There are two kinds of facts we need to have in order to plan an effective program for change. One has to do with the nature of the change process and the other with our own personal mental health practices. Both are dealt with below. Begin by testing yourself on these mental health facts. They may change the way you think about some phase of your life.

1. Mental health is marked by a zest for living, self-actualization, and self-realization and not a mere absence of mental disorder.   True False
2. If you're mentally healthy, you tend to conform to society.   True False
3. Once a person has a mental illness, he shouldn't be given a position of responsibility.   True False
4. With prompt and proper treatment, most patients admitted to a mental hospital can have partial or total recovery.   True False
5. The overwhelming majority of persons suffering from depression respond to treatment.   True False
6. Your psychological state can affect how long you live.   True False
7. Relationships with others can affect how long you live.   True False
8. One in 10 Americans suffers mental or emotional illness and requires professional help.   True False
9. Employees with emotional and mental problems detract from a company's ability to use manpower efficiently.   True False

ANSWERS
1. TRUE. Good mental health denotes more than the absence of mental illness, just as good physical health denotes more than the absence of physical illness.
2. FALSE. One of the major characteristics of self-actualizing people is that they don't confuse what the society happens to think is right with what *is* right. They may conform on many minor things, but on the big things they manage to keep free for their own choice. Self-actualizing people also report more peak experiences than people who are less self-actualizing.

3. FALSE. Although many people seem to think this way, especially in government positions, it has meant a tragic loss of talent.

4. TRUE. With greater understanding about emotional and mental problems, both the medical and behavioral science fields have developed diagnostic and treatment procedures to help a wide variety of problems. Early identification and proper treatment are often vital to recovery.

5. TRUE. There are many treatments for depression for those who can't shake it.

6. TRUE. Studies have shown that our psychological states can shorten life expectancy. There is, for example, an increased mortality rate among neurotic patients. One study describes a "predilection to death" among people whose lives had lost their meaning. Many researchers recommend avoiding unnecessary stress in order to reduce the incidence of disease and therefore prolong life.

7. TRUE. The ties that bind people together also apparently help them live longer, according to a nine-year study of nearly 7,000 Californians. The study showed that people who did not have strong social relationships were two to four and one-half times more likely to die. For those who stayed comparatively healthy it made little difference whether their social network was composed mainly of a spouse, friends, or an organization of some kind, as long as there were enough social contacts. The social factors seem somehow to influence general resistance or vulnerability to disease.

8. TRUE. Mental illness is a major problem in the United States.

9. TRUE. Often mental and emotional problems are a major drain on a company's productivity and efficiency. Some $20 billion are wastefully lost because companies have delayed developing effective mental health programs.

And now it might be well to look at some facts about ourselves.

TEST A: SOME POSITIVE MENTAL HEALTH PRACTICES

Below are listed some positive mental health practices that many people aspire to. Circle the *Yes* or *No* after each question to give yourself some idea of how you are doing in the areas. Later, you will have a chance to develop some plans in relation to some of those areas that you consider most important.

Are you mostly happy with your life?	Yes	No
Do you express your emotions in a constructive way?	Yes	No
Do you consistently work at and build good human relationships with those around you?	Yes	No
Are your relationships generally such that they enhance you and the other people with whom you are in contact?	Yes	No

Do you have some people whom you consider to be good friends and who consider you a good friend as well?	Yes	No
Are your relationships with other people generally meaningful and satisfying?	Yes	No
Do you usually work out your problems with others in an open and constructive way?	Yes	No
Do you contribute significantly to the enjoyment of your own life and to that of at least one other person?	Yes	No
Do you tend to let people you love and admire know how you feel about them?	Yes	No
Are you usually willing to share your feelings, emotions, hopes, and aspirations with people close to you?	Yes	No
Do you maintain a mentally healthy outlook on life most of the time?	Yes	No
Do you think pretty well of yourself and of your achievements most of the time?	Yes	No
Do you feel productive in your work or vocation?	Yes	No
Do you avoid negative put-down judgments about yourself?	Yes	No
When you are angry, do you express your feelings in a genuine yet constructive manner?	Yes	No
If you have a problem, do you feel free to seek assistance from your family or your friends, and, where necessary, secure professional help or counseling?	Yes	No
Do you feel a sense of purpose in life, that your life has meaning and direction?	Yes	No
Do you have some means of expressing your creativity in your job or through a hobby?	Yes	No
Do you spend enough time on the activities that you like the most?	Yes	No
Do your days come close to being used in the ways you would like them to be?	Yes	No
Do you feel you are in control of your life, rather than that your life decisions are out of your hands?	Yes	No
Do you face your daily tasks with pleasure and satisfaction rather than pain and boredom?	Yes	No
Do you feel active and involved enough in life?	Yes	No
Does love play an important enough role in your life?	Yes	No
Do you have enough caring in your life, you for others and others for you?	Yes	No

TEST B: SOME INCOMPLETE SENTENCES ON LIFE PLANNING

These incomplete sentences can help you think through some of the more central issues of your life. Later, your answers can be used to help you plan a program of improvement and change. Complete each one with the first thoughts that come into your mind.

My life is _____

_____

The best thing about my life is _____

_____

The worst thing about my life is _____

_____

More than anything, I want _____

_____

The things in life that have made me happiest _____

_____

The thing I would like different in my life _____

_____

TEST C: PRIORITIES AND GOALS

We tend to be busy doing trivial things in life. Then in our old age rocking chair we wonder why we didn't do more. A look at what our priorities are and how we're fitting them into our lives will help us avoid those rocking chair blues ("Oh, if I only had . . . .") later on.

Try putting your priorities down where you can take a good hard look at them. The five major priorities that I would like to see governing my life right now are:

1.
2.
3.
4.
5.

When I look at how I am allocating my time and energy, my five major priorities *appear* to be:

1.
2.
3.
4.
5.

Sometimes the lists don't match at all. And examining this data gives us an opportunity to see if we can't rearrange our time allocations with the priorities that we set for ourselves.

If there is a difference between what you would like and what actually is, then list what, if anything, you would like to do to bring about change.

What I would like to do is this:

_____

_____

TEST D: OUR RELATIONSHIPS WITH OTHERS

The quality of our relationships with others is important to our health and to the relationships of our potential as human beings.

Score yourself by which column most closely describes which relationship you have with your family, friends, and co-workers. Underline those areas that you would most like to improve. You can use this information later to begin a program of change.

	Excellent; needs no improvement	Needs some improvement	Not acceptable; needs major improvement
Mother	1	2	3
Father	1	2	3
Brothers and sisters	1	2	3
Husband	1	2	3
Wife	1	2	3
Children	1	2	3
Friends	1	2	3
Acquaintances	1	2	3
Neighbors	1	2	3
Boss	1	2	3
Work contacts	1	2	3

What steps can I take — both immediate and long-range — to improve those relationships that can be improved?

_____

_____

Many of us require professional help for dealing with acute emotional problems. The checklist below can help you decide whether you need to receive that help at this time.

Do you have bouts of uncontrollable anger?

Are you becoming suspicious of everyone, especially those near and dear to you?

Are you performing activities that are weird?

Are you frequently too tired or too keyed up to sleep, or even to think or function properly?

Do you have irrational crying fits?

Are you thinking seriously of suicide, murder, or sexual assaults?

Are you so nervous you need to take a pill when facing meetings or decisions or to get you through the day?

Do you feel as if you want to run away?

Are you so depressed you have no interest in your family or friends?

Do you have an uncontrollable compulsion to perform certain acts or rituals without knowing why?

Do you sometimes seriously wonder if you are losing your mind?

Are you becoming or are you already addicted to alcohol or other drugs?

Do you notice a decrease in your mental functioning, loss of memory, inability to think clearly?

Have you had a sudden or pronounced change in behavior?

If you answer yes to any of these questions, don't put off getting professional help. Discuss your problem with your doctor, who can help you determine if physical factors are causing your difficulties. If it is not physical, he or she can give you advice on whom to contact for further assistance. Or go to a clinic or community health center, or contact a local chapter of a mental health association for assistance. In many cities you can also dial hotlines for help with emotional problems, alcoholism, drug addition, or suicidal urges, etc. Many companies also provide confidential employee counseling services.

The important thing is not to accept severe depression, constant anxiety, or other mental symptoms as natural or necessary, but go to see a professional for help. If your problems don't require professional help, you can go on to Step Three.

Step Three. Find or Build a Supportive Environment

In the area of mental health especially, it is hard to go it alone. And there is really no reason to, since almost all of us are looking for many of the same things from our lives. Joy, happiness, and fulfillment, a chance to feel productive, wanted, and loved, are goals that are shared by many of us. To be sure, we have different ways of achieving them, but that doesn't hide the fact that our goals have a great deal in common and that there is a lot we can do to be supportive of one another.

The Lifegain support groups fulfill this function for many people. Others turn to family and friends, some to churches, or to the myriad of formal and informal groups that have become part of their lives.

Though there is a great deal of professional help available for people with mental health problems, some people tend to avoid or put off going to any of the psychologists, psychiatrists, and other practitioners trained to deal with mental illness, fearing that seeking such help is an admission of some grave weakness or limitation. If the truth were known, perhaps most of us could benefit from such help from time to time in our lives, if we would be mature enough not to be caught in the culture trap of having to do it alone.

There are thousands of self-help books written each year. If they aren't too simplistic, many of these have valuable ideas to offer. (See the annotated bibliography in the back of this book.) But remember, most of these ideas disappear if a supportive environment is not developed to maintain them.

Step Four. Put Your Own Plan Into Action

Your time is not forever. How many years do you have? And of those precious days and hours how many are you spending fulfilled, satisfied, happy; and how many in ways you don't like?

The purpose of this Lifegain program is to help you gain control of your life so that you can spend your time in the ways that you really want, and so you can have a better relationship with yourself and others as you go along.

In Step Two you analyzed your strengths and your weaknesses to see what you might want to work toward. Now you need to determine if these goals truly reflect your interests and values and whether you are willing to make them a priority. Write down the specific goals you want to work toward. Itemize them — 1, 2, 3 — so they are not floating, nebulous abstractions, but are straightforward, concrete, understandable points that can be frequently reviewed. Then next to each of these goals, write down some specific steps you can take to help you reach each of them.

Warning: Your biggest enemy may be your negative self encouraged by your negative culture. It is absolutely astounding how most of us manage to sabotage our own desires by throwing self-doubt, fears, inertia, and other obstacles in our way even when we want to do something. And often, because our culture has taught us to be that way, we are afraid of failure, of rejection, or of not enough reward for our efforts. A woman wants to be with people but doesn't want to go out alone. A man wants to talk to the

woman alone at the next table but is afraid of appearing foolish or being put
down. A person at the office feels some things there could be improved
that would make everybody happier and more productive, but never gets
around to talking it over and making the suggestion because "it just isn't
done around here."

To deal with this put-down aspect of ourselves, many of us have to overcome our own resistance to get moving. Perhaps two key questions to ask
yourself when you get to the point of sabotaging your own desire to do
something are: What are the potential rewards if I do it? What is the worst
thing that can happen if it goes wrong?

So often solutions toward a more satisfying life sound simplistic; the
answers seem so overly simple that you don't do them. The things that we
are discussing in this chapter have worked for many people. We urge you to
test some of them for yourself.

Self-realization is a lifetime task and a lifetime opportunity. To become all
that we are capable of being is a task that can never be fully achieved. To
have fully arrived is to stop growing, and to stop growing is a problem of
major proportions.

Making use of the facts that were developed in Step Two, we can now
begin to plan and implement our own individualized program for improvement, making use of a chart such as the one shown below. Since there are a
number of steps possible for each goal, each goal should be put on a separate
card.

Goal	Steps to Goal Achievement
To spend more time on my art	Schedule one hour each day
To improve my relationships with my parents	Discuss with them in a constructive way some of the problems that we may be having in our relationship

GETTING MOVING

Begin with the first step. Don't expect to do everything, at least not at first.
Seek help from others when you need it. Keep a sense of humor and perspective. As the poet Robert Frost said, "Everything will be all right if nothing
goes wrong with the lighting." He meant the sun and not our dining room
fixtures.

As you are working on your goals, there are some things to keep in mind:

Take one small step and begin to work on it first. Succeeding at small steps,
one at a time, has been proven more effective than trying to accomplish a
huge program at once and becoming discouraged.

Once you have made a decision, begin to sense your feelings and attitudes
as they are now, then make some small step in the direction you want to go.
If you want to improve your relationship with someone, pick up the phone
or write to them right now.

Make time for what you really want to do. Get up a half hour earlier (and go to bed a half hour earlier if necessary), shorten the time you spend on routine trivia, decrease the time you spend with television and magazines. (The national average for television watching is four hours a day — that's more than 7,000 hours a year!)

Vow to look at your successes, not your failures. Everyone who has ever tried anything has had whopping failures and mistakes. The trick is not to dwell on them but to look at them as one more experience of life. As the learned scholar Epictetus said in the second century A.D., "What disturbs men's minds is not events but their judgments on events."

Picture yourself as you want to be. If you want to be self-confident, think of yourself as self-confident. If you want to be articulate, picture yourself as articulate.

If you feel that you are not really doing the things you want to, explore some new interests that you have, or take up old interests that still excite you but that you dropped for awhile. Examine yourself for a sense of direction, one in which you would like to direct your energies, that will give meaning and substance to your life. Reevaluate the reasons you have given yourself for not doing things you would like to. Sometimes just stating the reason openly makes it seem less final and absolute.

IMPROVING RELATIONSHIPS WITH YOUR FAMILY AND FRIENDS

Try listening. Really listen to others: not with one eye on the television or your mind on what you're going to do tonight, but listen with both ears, with empathy, and with understanding.

Be as caring as you can be. Give the other person reassurance if he or she needs it. Even when you are asking people to change a behavior in some way, let them know you are asking because you care about them. Let people know you are on their side.

Try being noncompetitive. Don't feel you have to one-up the other person or prove your accomplishments to him or her. Let other persons enrich your knowledge and life with their experiences, and be willing to enrich their lives with what you have learned. But don't make the differences threatening.

Don't put down or be put down. As one workshop participant said: "Every time I go home I am surrounded by nagging remarks and negative feelings. Why do people have to be so negative?" She counteracted the problem by not asking for opinions and by purposely looking for something positive and complimentary to say to people, and found that it gradually had some effect, improving family relationships.

Talk things out. Don't keep bad feelings or frustrations bottled up. Talk about your feelings, your fears, your hopes, instead of always hiding your real self.

Put yourself in the other person's mind. Try to project yourself totally into what he or she is feeling and experiencing. This kind of increased empathy will bring you closer and prevent many problems from ever occurring.

Put transactional analysis to work. It shows you how to put "I'm okay, you're okay" into practice.

Appreciate differences. Don't fight them or be threatened by them. Be appreciative and understanding of a different background or interest.

Take responsibility for our own moods. Don't be a blamer. "If my husband paid more attention to me, I wouldn't be so depressed." "If my wife wouldn't nag so much, I wouldn't be so grouchy." Take responsibility for taking care of yourself and your moods.

HOW TO HANG ON WHEN THINGS GET OUT OF HAND

When you're furiously angry, frustrated, or despairingly disappointed, here are some ways mental health professionals recommend to get under control:

- Confront the problem when it's appropriate to do so.
- Do something strenuous and physical—tennis, golf, handball, a brisk walk. Lose yourself in the activity.
- Do something with your hands—knit, make bread, sand your boat, plant flowers. (Don't use power tools; it's dangerous when you're angry.)
- Listen to music, a record or a concert, classical or jazz; or dance; whatever relaxes you.
- Do some work—write checks, scrub the floor, trim the bushes, something that requires concentration.
- Talk to a friend. Tell him or her you're about to explode and why. Talk it out.
- Have some fun. Watch a funny movie, or call a friend who tells good jokes, or laugh at your own bad mood.

Step Five. Keep Track And Tune In

Most Lifegain participants find the best way to keep track is either by discussions in their group meetings, or if they do not meet regularly, to go over the questionnaires in Steps One and Two themselves and analyze whether they are making progress toward good mental health practices.

From time to time, take out the goals that have emerged from the tests you took in Step Two and from your initial plan in Step Four and review them. One Lifegain member keeps a card listing his major priorities in his wallet and reviews them regularly in relation to the ways he is spending his time and energy. Be sure you do this often so you don't run across your goals five or 10 years from now and find you haven't made any progress.

Another workshop group had members write postcards to themselves. "Dear Steve: Your goals were to spend more time on the pleasures you've been denying yourself and more time in conversation with your wife. How are you doing?"

If you have a problem with worrying about things, it sometimes helps to keep a diary so you can look back and see what happened to yesterday's worries.

Step Six. Reward Yourself And Have Fun

To have fun and to enjoy yourself is the center of sound mental health practice. Having good mental health makes it possible for you to enjoy youself and have fun. Conversely, having fun makes for good mental health. In fact, fun is so beneficial that Freud once remarked good mental health is enjoying both work and play.

Being more pleased with life is the major reward of getting along well with yourself and others. It makes you feel as if you belong, it makes you feel loved and appreciated, it makes you happy and satisfied with yourself, and it makes you feel you are living a full life. You find you're giving yourself a smile in the mirror every morning and a pat on the back every night for being able to lead a happy life.

Step Seven. Reach Out To Others

Good mental health by definition involves reaching out to others, helping others to achieve their goals or resolve problems with which they struggle.

As you proceed with your plan, many situations will occur in which you can encourage others in your family, at work, at school, among your friends, or in your community to work toward fulfilling their potentials.

As you make attempts to help others get along better, try to involve people in the solution of their own problems. Help them see ways to create success environments rather than environments where people tend to fail. Help them think in terms of cooperation instead of competition with their fellow workers, to search for win-win solutions. Support good mental health practices in others when you notice them. Reward people with recognition for a job well done. Tell a father when you think he is understanding of a son's problems. Let children know when you appreciate them. Give others support when they are trying to make changes, either in themselves or in community and government projects concerning mental health.

WE CAN WORK FOR A CARING COMMUNITY

There are many people just like us who are waiting for the same encouragement we're waiting for.

There is a lack of caring in our culture and of showing we care. You can begin to change that by reaching out and caring in your own circles, moving into more real relationships, taking the first steps to confronting the isolation, the nontouching that exists in our society.

People tend to think only of professionals helping others in mental health. But there is a vast reservoir of human to human interactions that can change the world around. One group tells a story of a rehabilitation center for discharged mental patients. It was staffed with a small number of professionals and had a very modest budget, yet the rehabilitation rate was high. The reason — Bessie, the jovial cook with a third-grade education who had no professional status at all. But she cared. Bessie rehabilitated more of the former patients than the rest of the staff combined.

We need more Bessies.

We can let others know we care, and we can encourage creativity, awareness, give others freedom to find their own sense of order and direction in life.

We can go even further — to concern for resolving conflicts between nations and races; to concern for bringing people together in groups to function harmoniously instead of with hostility.

To be tender, loving, and caring, human beings must be tenderly loved and cared for. You can teach caring and touching to your children, not only enhancing your children's lives now and in the future, but possibly helping to institute caring patterns that could continue beyond their lives and yours, for generations of cultures to follow.

So in mental health — in getting along with ourselves and others — we can, more than anywhere else, show the principles of Lifegain: We have the capacity to become creators rather than to be victims of our environments. We can change our lives and our cultures.

13 Making Our Health Resources Work for Us

Nowhere in the field of health and health planning are the norms of our present health culture more in conflict with reality and with intelligent common sense than in the ways in which we currently use and misuse our physicians and other medical resources.

We have some of the best trained medical personnel that have ever been available, and yet our use of such personnel is such that it often contributes to the very problems that their training was designed to overcome.

Picture John Robinson, an employee who has faithfully had his regular executive physical once a year for the past 15 years. John smokes, is overweight, and sedentary. Up until last year his yearly examination revealed no specific biometric symptoms. Last year it showed a slightly elevated blood pressure. His physician told him to watch it. This year he spent $25,000 for bypass surgery. John and his wife are, strangely enough, thanking their lucky stars for the wonders of medical technology.

John is like many other Americans who are very rightfully appreciative of the technology that helps them when in serious trouble. But unfortunately he is also like many of us in waiting until he is in serious trouble to realize that he, and not his doctor, is responsible for his health.

As physicians tell us time and time again, there is very little they can do compared to what we can do for ourselves. Drs. Donald Vickery and James Fries wrote in their recent consumer's guide to medical care (TAKE CARE OF YOURSELF, sponsored by Blue Cross/Blue Shield)*: "You can do much more than your physician to maintain your own good health and well-being. With the exception of those diseases which are prevented by immunizations, surprisingly few diseases can be prevented by the physician."

How you work with your doctor can be as important a factor in how long you live and how well you live as the other health practices we have been discussing.

Since it is actually a health practice, you should follow the same kind of program you did for the others, getting the facts and following a plan step-by-step.

*Reading, Ma: Addison-Wesley, 1976, page 5.

THE LIFEGAIN PROGRAM FOR WORKING WITH YOUR MEDICAL RESOURCES

Step One. Understand Your Own Culture

In this area we need to begin by raising the level of awareness about what is happening to us in relationship to our physicians and medical resources. We can see how we have been brainwashed into thinking certain things and adopting certain attitudes about doctors, hospitals, health costs, and medicine.

Are any of these things true of you and your friends? Check the statements that are true in your group.

It is a norm in one or more groups that I belong to:

☐ for people to follow faddish-type health recommendations and programs without checking their medical validity.

☐ for people to see their doctor instead of themselves as being in charge of their medical and health programs.

☐ for people to agree to important surgical or medical procedures without making certain that they get other independent medical opinions.

☐ for people to accept the first physican that they visit or who is recommended to them instead of shopping around for a physician.

☐ for people not to worry about health matters until something goes wrong.

☐ for people to believe that if they ignore the warning signs of illness it will go away.

☐ for men to believe that it is "sissy" or unmanly to worry about their health.

☐ for people to accept without question any medical advice that is given to them.

☐ for their personal physicians to be too busy dealing with illness-related problems to spend much time on preventive medicine.

☐ for people to be afraid to ask their physicians for complete, clear explanations of what is being medically recommended to them.

And just as in the Big Eight health practices, when you work with your doctor you have to understand there are culture norms that influence your view of the doctor and his view of you.

The norms and even mystique surrounding medicine are so strong that some people are actually frightened when they have to deal with the medical profession. Many terms are in Latin, much is not explained to the patient. Frequently medicines aren't labeled, so patients don't know what they're taking or what it's for.

We are part of a health care culture that encourages us to give up responsibility for our own health and then when there is a crisis to expect dramatic cures from all-knowing and curing doctors.

When we are treated, if we follow advice at all, we follow it without question. Our cultures tell us that the health care system is so complicated that it's OK not to understand it. The doctor, hospital, dentist, insurance company "always knows best."

Many people are so blindly dependent on their physicians that they don't even try to contribute anything when they meet with their physician. They are so in awe of their doctors that they often don't describe all the symptoms that are bothering them or give their own hunches as to what might be troubling them or might help them. I don't want to bother the doctor with that, some of them say.

Some physicians say at times people are so embarrassed or afraid to tell them their symptoms, or afraid of taking up their time, that the doctor doesn't get the complete picture and so makes a wrong diagnosis, or maybe takes much longer than necessary coming up with the best treatment.

How many times have you thought you might call your doctor, but then hesitated to because you were afraid to bother him with something that might not be important enough?

How many times have you taken a medicine without asking what it was supposed to do for you or what possible side effects there might be?

How many times have you agreed to an important medical or surgical procedure without really understanding how it was supposed to work or what alternative there might be?

We recommend that you don't get caught in these culture traps with your doctors. Instead, build a good working relationship with them. Respect their knowledge and what they can do, but become an important part of the team yourself.

And take the primary responsibility for your own health.

One of the tragedies of our illness-based culture is that many of us have given up our responsibility for our own health practices. Somehow we have created a medical system that robs us of responsibility for our own health and in so doing, sometimes robs us of our actual health as well.

With the most sophisticated and most expensive medical care in the world, we spend only a few moments a year with our physicians. All the rest of the time our health is up to us. We are in charge of our health practices day by day.

The good physician will not resent your becoming an active patient. He will not resent your asking questions. He will not feel threatened if you ask for a second opinion concerning controversial procedures. He will be happy to have you truly concerned about your body and your health.

Your doctor will be happy to have a patient who really cooperates.

Step Two. Get The Facts And Separate Fact From Fiction

You can begin to get the facts about effective use of medical resources and positive relationships with your doctor, by trying this True and False test. See how many myths you have been taking for truths.

1. Many medical problems can best be handled in the home.   True   False
2. Physicians should be in charge of our health.   True   False
3. When our company picks up our health bill, it doesn't cost us anything.   True   False
4. Doctors should not be bothered with your reporting of trivial aches, pains, and concerns.   True   False
5. You can usually save money by keeping old prescriptions on hand. You'll probably have the flu (or bronchitis, or whatever) again.   True   False
6. As a preventive measure, the complete annual physical is largely outmoded.   True   False
7. When in doubt, x-ray.   True   False
8. Complete multiphasic screening (lab tests including blood studies, x-rays, urinalysis, electrocardiogram) costs less and is the best way to detect problems that need immediate attention.   True   False
9. There is little need for adults to keep immunizations up with frequent booster shots.   True   False
10. If a drug does not require a prescription, it is a safe one.   True   False

These questions all touch on prevalent myths that influence our thinking about medical resources. Here are the answers:

1. TRUE. For acute medical problems you will probably need the hospital, but there are many lesser problems that are better off treated at home. Often the home atmosphere can be more therapeutic. Infection (particularly those due to *Staphylococcus*) is a constant problem in hospitals so it is not wise to remain in the hospital any longer than necessary.
2. FALSE. You are the best person to take charge of your own health. Learn to use the physician's skills when necessary, but don't overuse him. The final decisions about your health rest with you.
3. FALSE. The company spends money on illness costs that could be used for bonuses or salaries or other benefits.
4. TRUE. But whenever a truly important complaint or finding occurs, it is best to seek medical care without delay. These might be: running a fever for more than a week, finding a lump in the breast, losing weight suddenly without reason, coughing up blood.
5. FALSE. In the long run it may cost you a lot more. Some drugs are affected by heat and time. Also you might take the wrong one.
6. TRUE. The executive physical, often taking several days, is slowly being discontinued by the large corporations. Even though the "routine checkup" is no longer in favor, medical checkups *are* valuable, and are discussed later in this chapter.

7. FALSE. Although the amount of radiation in x-ray is small, it all adds up. Therefore, it is best to avoid x-raying whenever possible.

8. FALSE. Complete multiphasic screening (which performs 50 or more different tests) works quickly and often costs less, but experience over several years shows that few problems that need immediate treatment are found. Drs. Vickery and Fries comment: "Multiphasic screening procedures have become a means of mass reassurance. . . Screening is justified only for those individual tests which potentially detect important and treatable disease."

9. TRUE. With the increasing rarity of many diseases that once were epidemic, there is little need for continual immunizations in adult life. For many people, smallpox and diphtheria shots last for life. Flu shots are recommended only for older people and those with severe lung diseases.

10. FALSE. Over-the-counter drugs are not automatically safe and can be misused, sometimes with serious consequences. All drugs—if used in effective dosages—have the potential for side effects. Therefore manufacturers, to protect themselves, often recommend the smallest dosage feasible. The best thing to do is to try to learn something about the drugs you use or are likely to use, and use your educated common sense in treating yourself with them.

GIVE YOURSELF A CHECKUP—ARE YOU TAKING RESPONSIBILITY FOR YOUR OWN HEALTH?

Do you keep tuned in to your body so that you can be alert to possible body needs or danger signals?

Do you know the danger signals for serious illness?

Do you consistently assume full responsibility for your own health?

Do you know your medical history in detail, and do you keep a record of important facts?

Do you keep yourself informed about new health recommendations, separating fads and fictions from proven facts, and take them into account in your health-related decisions?

Do you know basic first aid for everyday problems and for emergencies?

Do you have basic emergency supplies in your home?

Do you keep track of immunizations and see that you and your children get all the necessary shots at recommended times? (Although dehabilitating diseases like polio have been virtually eliminated by mass immunization, continual alertness is needed to keep them in check. It is sobering to note that a good-sized portion of the population is *not* immunized against the six typical childhood problems—diphtheria, tetanus, polio, measles, rubella, mumps (24 percent to 44 percent of five to nine-year-olds and 30 to 50 percent of one to four-year-olds are not, depending on the diseases.)* You can do your part and protect your children by having them immunized during their first five years. After that, diphtheria and tetanus is recommended only every 10 years for life, with tetanus boosters only when a wound occurs five years after the last booster.

Do you have periodic checkups of your blood pressure and lungs?

Have you followed the recommendations for the improvement of your health that were given to you at the time of your last examination?

Have you learned how to do and do you conduct a periodic self-examination of your breasts?

Do you secure medical advice and assistance promptly when you need it?

Do you have a physician in whom you have confidence?

Do you make certain that you are fully informed about every aspect of your medical care?

Do you tell your physician your concerns, ask questions, express disagreement when you feel it, and ask for additional opinions when you are in doubt about a particular recommendation?

Do you have regular dental checkups, and have you taken the corrective measures that were recommended to you at the time of your last dental examination?

Are you alert to the signs of tooth or gum disease, and do you take steps quickly when such signs appear?

Do you read labels carefully?

When drugs or medicines are prescribed for you, do you check out the potential harmful effects that they might have on your body before taking them and discuss these effects with your physician?

Do you take only drugs or medicines that have been specifically recommended or prescribed for you?

Do you make certain that you don't mix drugs that can be harmful when taken in combination with one another, such as antidepressants and alcohol?

Do you know when *not* to run to the doctor?

Do you know what to do in the most common medical emergencies?

Do you know what medical problems you can treat at home and how?

If you are going to be in charge of your own health, if you are going to do a good job of taking your life in your own hands, you should have answered *yes* to all the questions above.

If you are going to become an active part of the medical team in charge of your own health, you must be active in working with your doctor. If you are to take the ultimate responsibility for your body and your health, that means you have to assume the responsibility for following the recommendations your doctor prescribes and for carrying out the lifestyle and health

*United States Immunization Survey, 1977, conducted by the Census Bureau.

habits that will give you total health and make you feel best. You will be in charge.

The beautiful thing about becoming an active responsible patient is that approaching the health care system as a partner usually gives you a feeling of self-confidence, of being in control. Partnership takes the mystery — and for many people, the fear — out of working with doctors, hospitals, insurance companies, and other parts of the system.

BEING YOUR OWN EARLY WARNING SYSTEM – A BODY CHECK

Part of total care of your car is using the check list in your owner's manual. Here's an owner's manual check list for your body.

Check any of the following problems that you have now:

☐ Sore or growth on the skin, lips, mouth, or tongue that doesn't seem to heal

☐ Any persistent itching that you can't explain

☐ Any enlarged lymph glands

☐ Moles that have changed color or size or become ulcerated or bleeding

☐ Development of a persistently hoarse voice

☐ Persistent difficulty in swallowing

☐ A constant cough

☐ Sputum streaked with blood

☐ Swelling of both ankles

☐ Unexplained dizzy spells

☐ Frequent serious nosebleeds

☐ Pain or burning on urination

☐ Blood in the urine

☐ Black, brown, or greenish urine

☐ Difficulty in starting to urinate

☐ A need to urinate much more frequently than in the past

☐ Frequent attacks of heartburn, indigestion, or abdominal pains

☐ Nausea or vomiting that has lasted more than a week

☐ Recent appearance of persistent constipation or diarrhea

☐ Blood in the stool or a tarry black color

☐ Sputum yellow-to-green in color, or reddish, or brown

☐ Loss of more than 10 pounds for no apparent reason

☐ Unexplained loss of appetite for a period of time

☐ Becoming very overweight

☐ Severe chronic fatigue

☐ Any swelling or lumps anywhere in the body

☐ Shortness of breath for no apparent reason, especially doing things that never bothered you before

☐ Swelling or persistent pain in the pelvic region

☐ Any genital discharge that is yellow, thick, bad smelling, or that has lasted more than a few days

☐ Persistent problems with sexual functions

☐ Bleeding after intercourse

☐ Bleeding between menstrual periods

☐ Bleeding that has begun again after menopause

☐ Pain in the breast not related to menstrual periods

☐ Lumps in the breast

☐ Puckering of the breast skin

☐ Any discharge from the nipples

☐ Nervous, irritable, or depressed spells

☐ Severe sleeplessness

☐ Crying jags

☐ A feeling of a nervous breakdown coming on

☐ Developing a sudden persistent, excessive thirst

☐ A squeezing or pressing feeling or a pain in your chest

☐ Yellow color to the skin or eyes

☐ Dimming or loss of vision

☐ Frequent earaches

☐ Running ears

☐ Sudden loss of hearing

☐ Head noises

☐ Dizziness

☐ Headaches that are extremely severe, return again and again, or are accompanied by nausea or vomiting or blurred vision

☐ Needing several drinks every day

☐ Frequently getting drunk

☐ Convulsions

☐ Frequent fainting

☐ Persistent numbness, loss of sensation of any part

☐ Loss of taste or smell

☐ Loss of strength or function, with dropping of things or stumbling

□ A serious pain that won't go away

□ Sweating or fever that keeps coming and going or has lasted for several weeks

□ Any symptom, even a sore throat, that persists or repeatedly returns and is not due to any obvious cause

If you had no checks, you scored very well on absence of illness. If you answered "yes" to any question, you should immediately make an appointment to see your doctor to discuss the symptom and have it checked further. You may find a temporary condition easily treated, or you may find the appointment was lifesaving.

UNDERSTAND MORE ABOUT MEDICINE

Though medicine is complex, you can understand more about it than you think. Ask questions of your doctor; take notes when you make a visit; if you don't understand what you are told, ask for more explanation. Look up medical words if you don't know what they mean. When your doctor uses a word and you don't know what it means, ask for a translation.

By breaking it down to its component parts, you can usually figure out the meaning of any medical word. A few samples: *itis* means inflammation, so arthritis means inflammation of a joint, carditis means inflammation of the heart. *Cranio* means skull, and *otomy* means hole, so craniotomy means making a hole in the skull, and tracheotomy means making a hole in the windpipe. *Hyper* means excess, so hyperthyroid means too much thyroid hormone. *Hypo* means deficiency or decrease, so hypothyroid means too little thyroid hormone.

And those fancy abbreviations need not be threatening. TLC only means tender loving care; BP means blood pressure; IM means intramuscular; RBC means red blood count.

Prescriptions, too, are not complex if you simply understand the language. Some of the key symbols:

prn	as needed
gtts	drops
mg	milligrams
od	right eye
os	left eye
ac	before meals
pc	after meals
qd	every day
qh	every hour
b.i.d.	two times a day
t.i.d.	three times a day
q.i.d.	four times a day

Be sure you are not antiphysician. Your doctor is there to help you. You gain nothing by being antagonistic or cynical.

And most important, when your doctor gives you advice, follow it. If you are given medicine, take it. Studies show as many as 60 percent of people go to a physician and then ignore the advice, don't fill a prescription, don't take the medicine properly, or don't finish taking the medicine after they buy it. (If a treatment does not seem to be working or is causing a side effect, call your doctor, who can then alter the instructions. Do not stop taking medicines on your own without letting your doctor know.)

THE FAMILY AS A SUPPORT GROUP

The more you can acquaint your family with what you are trying to do, and the deeper you get them involved in examining their attitudes and behavior in regard to medical resources, the better off you and they will be. It stands to reason that a coordinated family health plan, with a doctor who knows all the family, will work to the best advantage of everybody. Except for times when a specialist or subspecialist is needed by individuals in the family, you can all use the same physician.

Air your feelings about medicine, hospitals, and doctors with your family and find out how they feel. Then together you can provide a supportive atmosphere that will help all of you practice preventive medicine at home and approach doctor and hospital visits with a responsible attitude.

Your Lifegain support group can give you further help in making the changes you want.

Look over the facts and ask yourself about your desire to change your present relationship with the medical care system.

Are you satisfied with your present physician?	Yes	No
If not, do you have a commitment to change?	Yes	No
Are you satisfied with your own attitude and behavior in relation to your doctor and other medical resources?	Yes	No
Do you need to know more about the medical resources in your area?	Yes	No
Do you need to know more about medical costs?	Yes	No
Have you shared any of these commitments with family, friends, or others?	Yes	No

Step Four. Decide For Yourself

Develop a plan. Decide what you'd like to be doing for your own health.

A number of areas your plan might cover are discussed below. Read them over and see which ideas you would like to include in your own special plan for working with your medical resources.

THE LIFEGAIN MEDICAL CHECKUP

We are recommending an entirely new kind of medical checkup.

With this checkup you get the usual medical tests that you need — blood pressure (you may have taken it yourself at home but the doctor will want to check on it), the TB skin test or X-ray (every three to five years, or yearly if you have been exposed to TB), an annual Pap smear for women, glaucoma test (after 40 years of age if there is a family history of it). Your doctor may advise additional blood tests, urinalysis, etc., for special reasons, and immunization shots.

For children, the following timetable is generally recommended:

2 months: Diphtheria, whooping cough, tetanus (DPT) — first shot; polio — first shot

4 months: DPT — second shot; polio — second shot

6 months: DPT — third shot; polio — third shot

12 months: Measles, mumps, rubella

18 months: DPT booster; polio booster

5 years: DPT booster; polio booster

After this, diphtheria and tetanus every 10 years, additional tetanus if needed for a wound and if it happens 5 years after the last booster.

You may also want to include another element in your medical checkup — an in-depth conference with your doctor so the two of you together can analyze your current health habits, review your progress in the Big Eight areas, and make decisions about any changes you could make in your health practices to increase even further your enjoyment of life and your life expectancy.

As a preliminary to this conference you should make a list of any symptoms or problems you have that you wish to talk over with the doctor. Think not only about the early warning signals, but also about personal problems you might have hesitated to discuss before. Include family problems, work problems, sex problems, and other areas of stress. You should also bring in your medical history checklist if the doctor does not already have this information. Be sure to tell your doctor about any prescription or nonprescription medications you take on a regular basis, whether tranquilizers, sleeping pills, pain pills, diet pills, headache remedies, antidepressants, laxatives, antacids, hormones, pain relievers, antihistamines, decongestants, stimulants, birth control pills, vitamins, minerals, or others.

The most significant difference in the Lifegain checkup is your conference with the doctor about specific risks you might have and how you can improve your health habits to reduce those risks and improve your life.

You will want to discuss the amount of exercise you get; what you do, how long, how often, and whether it is sufficient to strengthen your cardiovascular system.

If you smoke, you should discuss what you smoke and how much.

You will want to discuss how much stress you are presently undergoing and whether it is affecting your sleep, your work, or your health. If stress is a problem at present, talk about some ways for you to handle it.

You will want to discuss your weight, whether it is the best weight for you, and if not, what changes should be made.

You will want to discuss your nutrition in general. Tell your doctor what you eat, especially foods you eat in large amounts. Discuss how much coffee, tea, and cola you drink; how much sugar and sweets you use; what you typically eat for your meals. Outline what vitamin and health food supplements you take.

You will want to discuss the alcohol you drink and how much, whether you go on drinking binges, whether you need a drink to go to sleep, whether your work or family life are ever affected by your drinking.

You will want to discuss if you are taking any drugs, including tranquilizers, alcohol or other addictive drugs, marijuana or cocaine, and how often.

You will want to discuss whether you practice automobile safety or drive when you have been drinking, whether you are exposed to dangerous situations or toxic materials at home or in your job.

You will want to discuss if you have had any recent important changes in your life, in sports, job, marriage, or whether you have changed any health habits drastically.

You will want to tell the doctor what pets you have, for they are sometimes disease carriers.

You will want to discuss any depression, irritability, hostility, or other emotional problems you are having, or if you're having trouble sleeping or getting along with other people.

You will want to discuss any sexual problems you are having, physical or emotional.

Play it straight with your doctor, for your health's sake.

Plan specific goals in any area where you or your doctor believe you need change: how to change your diet, how much weight to lose, what kind of exercise to do, how to stop smoking, etc.

An effective technique is to have everyone in the family see the doctor during the same week. Then at home you can talk about the results from your checkups and what programs you each have been recommended to follow. You can share ideas with each other on how you will make changes, make plans to have some fun doing it, and support each other during the changes.

Bob and Linda Scott and their children did it and found it completely changed their ideas about health. Said Bob, "I feel for the first time I'm really in charge of my health. I now have a physician I can, for the first time, relate to."

The Scotts frequently have family meetings to go over their programs to see how much progress they're all making.

Mary Steinway, her husband Bill, and their two sons also switched to this type of checkup. Before each examination they would look over the body checklist to remind themselves of any symptoms to report to the doctor, and they would retake the health practices survey, norm indicator, the 72-hour test (see Chapter 3), and the life expectancy test.

"It was marvelously supportive to all of us," Mary reports. "And we were having more fun with our lives. With the conferences we really felt in partnership with our doctor. A machine wasn't just blooping out standard instructions to the average middle age, middle weight, middle height, middle American, middle healthy patient. We were getting advice specifically geared to our needs, our lifestyle, our background, our desires, our risks, by someone who knew and cared about what we were doing."

Try it and see what it can do for your family.

IF YOU'RE LOOKING FOR A DOCTOR

There are many kinds of physicians — generalists or primary care doctors (like your family doctor or internist), specialists (like surgeons, psychiatrists), and subspecialists (like cardiologists, neurologists). Some practice alone, some in groups. Some are paid on a fee-for-service basis; some offer a prepayment plan similar to an insurance policy. There are also a wide variety of medical facilities — clinics, hospitals, emergency rooms, convalescent homes. How do you find what you want for your needs?

We can offer a few guidelines that will help you in making your choice of physicians:

- A generalist can determine the nature and severity of your problem and help you decide on whether or not you need a specialist and what kind.
- If you have determined what your particular problem is, a subspecialist in that area will most likely be best for you.
- If you are consulting a specialist, see if he has completed his boards in that specialty.
- Talk to your friends about the office practices of their doctors before deciding on yours. Make an informal survey among your friends to find out which doctors are interested in preventive medicine, which ones listen carefully.
- While seeing different doctors each time you need one works medically just about as well as seeing the same one, most of us want to build a relationship with someone who will be so important in our times of need.
- In most instances, the type of physician is not as important as the individual person.
- Having the same physician see everyone in the family will probably result in a better understanding of the individual members than if they went to separate doctors.
- Don't judge a doctor by the looks of the office.

- Don't expect house calls—very few doctors make them these days, except in cases where it is necessary for the comfort of the terminally ill. It's probably better that they don't. It would only add to the expense, and much of the technology that is available in an office would not be available in a home visit.

Give Your Doctor a Checkup. Does your doctor:

☐ Do a complete medical history at some point, asking many specific questions about your past health and your family's?

☐ If you are a woman, do a pelvic examination and a Pap smear? Check out any suspicious lumps in the breast that you have found in your monthly self-examination?

☐ Keep records and consult them at each visit?

☐ Measure your blood pressure at least once a year and tell you what he finds?

☐ Ask you about your eating habits and whether you exercise and whether you smoke or drink, and how much, and give you advice about these things when he should?

☐ Refer you to other specialists or call in a consultant when advisable?

☐ If a specialist, is he board certified?

☐ Go to meetings, read journals, participate in continuing education programs?

☐ Do any patient education such as giving out literature or recommending books?

☐ Have someone to cover for him on days or evenings off and during vacations?

☐ Take telephone questions to save you making an office visit?

☐ Have a helpful attitude, so you feel you can discuss anything with him, including sexual or emotional problems?

☐ Treat you as a participant in your own health care rather than putting you down for any opinions you might have?

☐ Encourage you in things you want to try such as improving your diet, breast feeding, exercising?

☐ Give you a complete diagnosis and explanation of any condition you might have so that you understand it?

☐ Explain the reasons for any special tests or treatments, and report the results to you?

☐ Explain what medicines he prescribes and tells you of any side effects to watch for?

☐ Have prescriptions labeled as to contents?

☐ Generally get good results with his treatments?

☐   Spend enough time with you, giving you a chance to explain completely
     any problems that you might have?
     Look over the questions you answered "no" to, and discuss them with
your doctor at your next visit.

WHEN YOU HAVE TO TAKE MEDICINES

Drugs can alleviate pain, reduce symptoms, save lives. Misused, they can do
just the opposite, adding to human suffering and even causing death. It is
essential, therefore, to know what drugs and medicines we are putting into
our bodies, what effects they have on us, and what the benefits should be
from taking them.
     Here are 16 rules to make sure medicines don't cause you more problems
than they help.

   Use medicines properly. Take exactly as directed. Don't stop taking a drug
      when you begin to feel better unless your physician says to. Often any-
      thing less than the full course of treatment may prevent the medicine
      from completely correcting the condition.
   When you have a prescription filled, use it. An amazing number of people
      spend time and money obtaining medicines and never take them.
   Make sure you really need the medicine. According to an article in *Science*,
      many doctors write prescriptions simply as ways to end an office visit.
      Don't encourage your doctor to give you medicines you don't need. Just
      because you go to your doctor with a problem doesn't mean you need
      medicine.
   Find the causes of your problems. You may spend hundreds of dollars on
      sleeping pills for years and then find it's too much coffee or alcohol that
      is keeping you awake. Coughing? Don't buy lozenges, give up cigarettes.
      Constant cold? Maybe you really have an allergy.
   Tell your doctor if you are not responding to a medicine. If this is the case,
      it may be necessary to change the treatment plan.
   Tell your doctor and your pharmacist to label as to contents. Know
      exactly what your medications are. The information can be invaluable
      when you change physicians or move to another locality. And in emer-
      gency situations, immediate identification of a drug from a label may be
      lifesaving.
   Read package inserts. The leaflet inside the package may tell you of pos-
      sible side effects, most effective treatment plans, any contraindications
      to taking the medicine.
   Ask your doctor questions about your drug prescription. What is the name
      of the drug and what is it supposed to do? What side effects should you
      be especially alert for and report? Are there any conditions in which the
      drug is unsafe? How often should the drug be taken, before or after
      meals, for how many days? Should the prescription be refilled and under

☐ Spend enough time with you, giving you a chance to explain completely any problems that you might have?

Look over the questions you answered "no" to, and discuss them with your doctor at your next visit.

WHEN YOU HAVE TO TAKE MEDICINES

Drugs can alleviate pain, reduce symptoms, save lives. Misused, they can do just the opposite, adding to human suffering and even causing death. It is essential, therefore, to know what drugs and medicines we are putting into our bodies, what effects they have on us, and what the benefits should be from taking them.

Here are 16 rules to make sure medicines don't cause you more problems than they help.

Use medicines properly. Take exactly as directed. Don't stop taking a drug when you begin to feel better unless your physician says to. Often anything less than the full course of treatment may prevent the medicine from completely correcting the condition.

When you have a prescription filled, use it. An amazing number of people spend time and money obtaining medicines and never take them.

Make sure you really need the medicine. According to an article in *Science*, many doctors write prescriptions simply as ways to end an office visit. Don't encourage your doctor to give you medicines you don't need. Just because you go to your doctor with a problem doesn't mean you need medicine.

Find the causes of your problems. You may spend hundreds of dollars on sleeping pills for years and then find it's too much coffee or alcohol that is keeping you awake. Coughing? Don't buy lozenges, give up cigarettes. Constant cold? Maybe you really have an allergy.

Tell your doctor if you are not responding to a medicine. If this is the case, it may be necessary to change the treatment plan.

Tell your doctor and your pharmacist to label as to contents. Know exactly what your medications are. The information can be invaluable when you change physicians or move to another locality. And in emergency situations, immediate identification of a drug from a label may be lifesaving.

Read package inserts. The leaflet inside the package may tell you of possible side effects, most effective treatment plans, any contraindications to taking the medicine.

Ask your doctor questions about your drug prescription. What is the name of the drug and what is it supposed to do? What side effects should you be especially alert for and report? Are there any conditions in which the drug is unsafe? How often should the drug be taken, before or after meals, for how many days? Should the prescription be refilled and under what circumstances? Should certain foods or activities or other medications be avoided while taking the medicine?

Don't keep old medicines. Any time a label is missing, a medicine turns color, is congealed or more concentrated, has started to crumble, or smells like vinegar, throw it out immediately. Always discard medicines on their expiration date.

Watch for side effects and allergic reactions. It is estimated that each year over 200,000 Americans die and many more — over 600,000 — are hospitalized because of adverse drug reactions. With any drug there is always the chance of a side effect.

Always tell a new physician of past drug reactions, even if they are mild. The next one may be more severe.

Warning signs of drug reaction: fever; fatigue; nausea and vomiting; wheezing or shortness of breath; inflammation of the eyelids and reddening of the eyes; skin rash, itching, or hives; blood in the urine; an agitated or upset emotional state; diarrhea or constipation. Call your doctor if you are taking medicine and any of these symptoms occur.

Beware of mixing medicines. Antacids, for example, can interfere with the action of tetracycline. Sedatives can counteract antidepressants. Nose drops can counteract high blood pressure pills. Antacids or Kaopectate can counteract digitalis.

Some drugs enhance other drugs, for example, aspirin and sulfa drugs, can enhance the effect of oral hypoglycemic pills or anticoagulants.

Don't drink alcohol when you are taking drugs. Alcohol can change the metabolism of many drugs and alter their effects. It can add to the depressant affect of tranquilizers on the central nervous system. Alcohol plus a barbiturate, for example, can kill you.

Ask your doctor if there are any foods you shouldn't eat. Some foods can be deadly combined with certain medicines. Great caution should be used with certain drugs that can produce side effects with certain foods. Though they are seldom used, it is well to check with your doctor, for they could kill you. Some foods, while not harmful in themselves, spoil the effect of certain medicines. Milk, for example, will keep tetracycline from working as it should.

Ask about cigarettes. If you must smoke, note that there are other drugs in addition to nicotine and tar that can be harmful. Some mint cigarettes contain atropine and scopolamine that affect the nervous system. And nicotine itself interferes with some medicines.

If you take an antibiotic, ask your doctor if you may also have a preparation of *Lactobacillus acidophilus* (Brand names: DoFus, Bacid or Lactinex). It will put back into the body the good germs that have been killed off by the antibiotic when it killed the bad germs and help prevent diarrhea, vaginal yeast infections, fungus infection, and irritability. Also, when an antibiotic is given to you, always finish the full amount. Otherwise, hidden lingering infection can start up again.

*Don't use over-the-counter medicines for long periods to control bother-
some symptoms.* They can cover up serious problems themselves. Using
throat lozenges for weeks to treat a sore throat, for example, can mask
a serious infection. Aspirin can cause stomach bleeding.

WHEN YOU HAVE TO GO TO A HOSPITAL

The time to choose the hospital you need is not when you are ill but long
before. Look into the facilities in your area and make your choices before
you actually need the services of a hospital.

In choosing a medical facility you will want one that offers primary care
close by — an emergency room, clinics, or doctor's office where you won't
need a referral. And you will want to be able to get easily to a second care
facility — a hospital with its specialists and subspecialists.

The hospital may be a private or community hospital or a public hospital
(like a VA hospital or county health unit). It may be a teaching hospital
associated with a medical school. These usually have excellent technical
resources, though the quality of personal relationships is variable.

Determine the nearest hospital to you that has an outpatient or emergency
room. Then if you are faced with a crisis and cannot reach your doctor, you
can go to the emergency room.

Remember, hospitals are expensive and are geared to handle crisis. Don't
use them as a place to rest, or for routine tests that can be done elsewhere.

Even if you have to go to the hospital you can still retain some control
over your own health. You can check backgrounds before choosing a surgeon. Obtain recommendations from other doctors and nurses you know and
confirm that the doctor does your particular operation frequently. (You do
not want a surgeon who does an operation only occasionally.) And make
sure he is on the staff at a good hospital.

Have your doctor explain the benefits and risks of the surgery and of
possible alternative treatments. Don't push a doctor into performing
unneeded surgery.

If there is any doubt in your mind whether you need surgery, get a second
opinion, especially for hysterectomy, gall bladder, hemorrhoids, or removal
of tonsils. Some Blue Cross plans and some other health plans will cover
charges related to a second opinion.

What To Do To Decrease Complications And Help You Heal Faster. Even a
simple step like having plenty of rest and eating very nourishing foods for
the weeks preceding an operation can make a difference.

If you are a smoker, stop smoking several days before surgery. If you
usually drink large amounts of alcohol, cut down before entering the
hospital.

If you have had a recent cold or other respiratory infection, postpone
elective surgery. If there is time, have infected teeth treated or pulled.

Discuss with your doctor chronic diseases, allergies, or any medicine you take. It may be necessary to adjust the dosage of some medications before surgery. If you have a chronic disease, have been taking cortisone or ACTH, are allergic to penicillin or other drugs, or if you have sickle cell anemia or other blood problems, you should inform both the anesthesiologist and the surgeon.

Some doctors recommend taking vitamin and mineral supplements before and after surgery. Several surgeons we talked to said the differences in recovery with certain vitamins and minerals can be quite significant, that wounds and broken bones heal faster, and that there is a decrease in the risk of postsurgical blood clots and emergency bleeding.

Another lifesaver within your control is exercise. Even while flat on your back in bed you can contract the muscles in your toes, feet, and legs, alternating squeezing and releasing as many times as you can, several times a day. And as soon as your doctor says you can, sit up and walk. This not only helps you heal faster but also helps prevent dangerous blood clots from forming in the leg veins.

You can also yawn, deeply and frequently. This superinflates the lungs, helping to clear bronchial secretions and prevent pulmonary complications that often occur after surgery.

Getting Along With Your Doctor In The Hospital.   Doctor visits in the hospital are brief because there are usually many patients to be seen, so make those visits as productive as possible. Have a prepared list of questions ready when your doctor stops by your room each day.

Although legally you are now allowed to see your chart and have access to all your medical records, it is very difficult to do so. And chances are you won't understand the medical terminology and abbreviations or be able to read the handwriting, so it's more satisfactory to ask your doctor to explain procedures that will be done and medicines you will be taking. This also gives you an extra check on medications to help ensure against the mistakes that occasionally happen.

There are other ways to protect yourself in the hospital. Tell the nurse or doctor if your sleeping pill isn't adequate, if your bowels don't move, and if you have any adverse reaction to medicines or treatments.

Step Five. Keep Track And Tune In

KEEP YOUR OWN MEDICAL FILE

Among your regular household files, set up one for medical records for yourself and your family. Include records of immunizations, diseases each has had, allergies, operations done, blood type, and any other pertinent data such as readings of high blood pressure, high cholesterol, or high triglycerides in the blood. It is helpful to your doctor to bring this history in with you on the first or any early visit.

YOUR FAMILY MEDICAL HISTORY

What are the present ages of your parents, or ages at death and causes of death?

Have you ever been told you had any of the following diseases: High blood pressure, diabetes, alcoholism, heart disease, stroke? Have any of your close relatives had those diseases?

Mark all of these on a chart like the following (Table 1). Show this chart to your doctor if he hasn't already gathered these facts.

TABLE 1. Family Medical History

	YOURSELF	GRANDPARENTS	MOTHER	FATHER	SIBLINGS	CHILDREN
Alcoholism						
Cancer						
Diabetes						
Allergies						
Heart trouble						
High blood pressure						
High cholesterol						
High triglycerides						
Depression, other mental illness						
Stroke						
Ulcers						
Weight problem						
Hereditary diseases						

Step Six. Reward Yourself And Have Fun

You reward yourself by improving your health and saving your money.

It is a lot better going to a physician in whom you have confidence and whom you have chosen freely for well thought out reasons. Having such trust in your physician is a reward in itself.

Going to the doctor only when you really need to and taking primary responsibility yourself will cut down your medical expenses. The first time you skip the annual executive-type "complete" physical, figure out what you have saved and buy yourself a treat.

Step Seven. Reach Out To Others

We'll all be helping our doctors by taking responsibility for ourselves. One of the major problems doctors have is that people think they can do anything. Then, when things don't go right, they feel terribly depressed. You can add immeasurably to their mental health by admiring them for the right things — their medical knowledge and expertise — but not expecting them to do the preventive job that you can best do yourself.

And you'll be helping doctors achieve a much more reasonable workload. Doctors are known to be overworked, even as patients are overdoctored. Getting the picture in balance will be a help to us all.

BE LESS THAN "PATIENT"

Think of yourself in relation to medical services as a consumer rather than as a "patient." By being reasonably knowledgeable and skillful in taking care of yourself, by being unafraid to ask questions and to make comparisons, by respecting your doctor's superior knowledge and experience, you can work to make the most of his or her skills for the benefit of your good health.

14 Lifegain in Your Organization or Community

It's tragic to think that the organizations and communities that we have created to better our lives are in fact serving to destroy us. Without our realizing it, they often act as counterforces to our personal efforts to gain better health. Fortunately, it doesn't have to be that way. It is possible for us to change the health cultures of our organizations and our communities, and a great many people are doing exactly that.

If you are a secretary, the president of a company, a student, a professor, an administrator, a town councilman, the head of a youth program, the wife of the mayor; if you are a union member, a member of the Chamber of Commerce, a clergyman, a church member; if you work on an assembly line, repair duplicating machines, write advertising copy, or run a dance studio, wherever you are in an organization, you can use the Lifegain system to help turn things around toward health rather than illness.

A number of people have already done so.

Martha, an elementary school teacher, was taking a graduate course in the evenings at a nearby college. She learned about the Lifegain system in her class and applied it to her elementary school. She was surprised at how soon she had the whole school—teachers, students, and parents—interested and involved in changing their health culture.

Martin, the president of a large manufacturing corporation, was concerned about the high toll in lives, absenteeism, and illness cost of the destructive health practices in his company. He determined that before he retired, he would make his company the healthiest in the country. Applying the Lifegain system, within a few months large numbers of people throughout the company were involved in understanding, identifying, and changing their own health practices and the health practices of the entire company.

An organization or a community that is contributing to poor health, shortened lifespans, high medical costs, really can turn itself around from a lifeloss to a lifegain culture. Whether it is a school, a business, an office, a store, a union, an agency, a hospital, or a community, there is a systematic, workable process through which you can help that organization change itself into a health supporting culture. The life-draining pull of the organization can be transformed into a life sustaining, health supporting force.

THE LIFEGAIN HEALTHY COMMUNITY SYSTEM

A number of organizations and communities are already at work on bringing about change. In Oliverea, New York, one of the largest and most successful residential camps in the world, the Frost Valley YMCA Camp, has made wellness and positive health the major focus of its camping program. What is more, the methods and materials that it has developed have been successfully introduced in a great many other camps throughout the country. The summer camping program has been so successful, in fact, that Frost Valley's school based environmental programs have also adopted wellness as one of their major emphases.

In Denver, Colorado, one of the most prestigious hospitals in the west, the Swedish Hospital System, has developed its own Wellness Center from which it distributes the Lifegain programs to companies, school systems, and other hospitals and health care agencies.

The Samaritan Hospital System of Phoenix, Arizona, which provides most of the hospital services in the Phoenix area, has also introduced its own culture based wellness program, making use of many of the ideas that you are reading about in this book. It has introduced the program to all of its employee groups as a prelude to implementing a broad community based program.

In Pawtucket, Rhode Island, a whole community is working together to change its health cultures. This program, which has just received a major long-term grant from the National Institute of Health, will provide one of the first carefully controlled longitudinal studies of the ability of people in communities to successfully modify their health cultures on a sustained basis.

In Stevens Point, Wisconsin, a university based program is bringing about positive changes in both the university and in the community. Both students and townspeople have reacted with enthusiasm.

Toward A Healthy America

One of the most encouraging signs of all is that the prestigious national coalition of health professionals, sports figures, and government and business leaders, known as Healthy America, has just adopted the Lifegain healthy community system as its major vehicle for community and organizational health promotion. As a result, plans are now being readied for a broad national effort backed by some of America's leading foundations, hospitals, corporations, and communities.

Who, Me? A Whole System?

Even if you are the newly hired cashier in a supermarket or a house bound mother of three children, you can take the health promoting principles you have already begun to put into use for yourself and place them in a workable structure for their use with an entire organization.

It is hard work, but it's fun, gratifying, and satisfying.

HOW YOU CAN USE THE LIFEGAIN SYSTEM

It is really not so difficult to change an organization or community as you might think. There are four main phases in the change process (Fig. 1).

Phase I. The Start-Up involves obtaining leadership commitment, developing volunteer and task forces, analyzing and setting goals.

Phase II. Involvement introduces the possibility of change. Workshops are held for everyone who wants to participate.

Phase III. Installing Change involves the day to day activities of both the individual and the organization. It includes individual self-help programs, Lifegain general and specialized support groups, and special task force programs.

Phase IV. Sustaining Change consists of evaluating what you have done, finding and achieving ways to extend the program to others, and keeping the good things going.

Phase I. Start Up

Keeping the above process in mind, the first step is to develop an informed awareness on the part of key organizational or community leaders. Fortunately this is not as difficult as it might at first appear. As we have seen, economic costs of our present lifeloss system are such that many if not most leaders are already alarmed by them. The human costs are even greater — there is hardly a person not affected.

In developing this informed awareness, you can start at the top or at the bottom. It is frequently easiest to begin by getting a commitment from the president, manager, mayor, governor, the director — whoever is in charge of the group you wish to influence. They often are the ones with the power to assign money and time, to designate personnel to do tasks, to set policies and make use of communications systems. Another way is to start from the bottom. Sometimes leaders will respond if enough people ask for change. It is a matter of getting a large enough and vocal enough group together and letting the leadership know how you all feel.

Suppose *you* are the leader. Then you have a head start, but you will still need to get commitment from others — the board of directors, the faculty leaders, the trustees. You need to get commitment also from the hidden leaders — the schoolyard leaders, the inner circle at the church, those who are looked up to. Whose advice is sought? Who is listened to? If you can get the

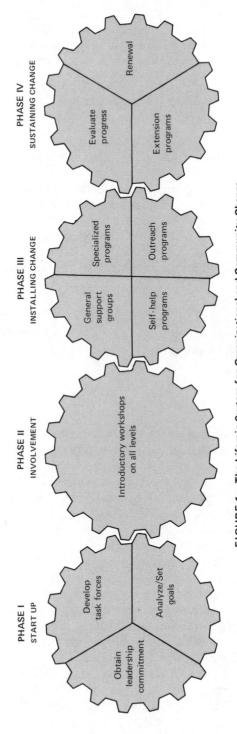

FIGURE 1. The Lifegain System for Organizational and Community Change.

commitment of these people, you will have a better chance of getting your program off the ground, for their support can often have a snowballing effect on the rest of the group.

The important thing is to get past the wall of skepticism and apathy and to get past blame placing. You focus on what can be done, rather than on the wrong ways people have tackled all this in the past. This does not mean ignoring the negatives—it is important to analyze what is wrong and know what you are dealing with. But because you are focusing on results, not blame, you are more likely to get something done and to get the support you need.

We have found that most organization leaders are receptive to the kind of ideas expressed in the Lifegain program. If your organization does not have that kind of welcome mat out, there are still ways to get started. The chief trick is to avoid the emotional reactions that can shut off new ideas and new understandings. No matter what is wrong in the organization, in approaching a leader about a new idea, avoid placing blame. You can present the problem as a mutual problem or as a problem you see being influenced by many people. This is quite different from confronting the company with a "You're-doing-things-wrong-and-we're-not-going-to-stand-for-it-any-more" attitude. Identify yourself as part of the culture that has been supporting the negative norms and instead of blaming others, point out the sad truths of the culture traps we are all caught in.

As one starter, you might show the Lifegain organizational support indicator (described later) to the boss, and ask if it might be used to do a survey of how people feel. Surveys like these can be motivating forces sparking interest in a health practices program, and later they can be used in measuring progress.

Or you might give a copy of this book to your boss with a covering letter offering to work on any planning committee that might be established if he or she were interested in trying these ideas in your organization.

When you talk to a leader in a business organization, think of increased profits as a place to start the conversation. If you are approaching a religious organization, an approach might be the relationship of sound mind and body to spiritual growth; or, you might stress the potential of increased church membership that the new program might bring.

The purpose in starting from the other person's interest is not to be manipulative but to find mutual individual and group goals. Changes that help individuals' health practices will be much more lasting if they also contribute to the goals of the organization or community.

THE KIND OF COMMITMENT YOU WANT

You want more than lip service. If you get "Sounds fine, go ahead and do it and let me know how you make out," that's one step. But do your best to get a further tangible commitment—budgeting of money and time for the program, setting up of meetings, or communicating to the rest of the organization that the president of the company, the minister of the church, the superintendent of the school system is personally committed to the project.

Your enthusiasm will help get this kind of commitment. It can spark the other person's enthusiasm. But back your enthusiasm with facts — about the present health of the organization, about the Lifegain program, about the results that might be possible. You don't have to be comprehensive — but you need enough information to show that something can be done.

GETTING ON WITH THE PROGRAM

Once you have the go-ahead, it is time to begin to involve the rest of the organization or community in the plan. This can be accomplished through a letter or a series of meetings announcing the purpose of the program and asking for volunteers to help get it underway. Sometimes volunteers can be recruited by personal calls. In one organization more than 35 per cent of the people volunteered for leadership!

The volunteers will need to be given a full understanding of the program so that it becomes theirs rather than something imposed from outside. Key leaders from the volunteer group can then be selected or elected to form a central Lifegain Committee. This committee is responsible for overall program, provides leadership, and each member of the committee assumes responsibility for a specific health practice area, such as exercise, smoking, nutrition, alcohol, etc. Each one of these committee leaders then establishes his or her own task forces which provide the leadership in the particular health area assigned to them and also establishes specialized support groups in those areas.

Sometimes task forces can also be established to deal with specific areas of concern, such as family participation, school participation, media participation, etc.

The most important task of the leadership group is to make certain that its own members are fully involved in the Lifegain program. In this way they can model the program for other people and also build up their own commitment and enthusiasm. It is unlikely that a leadership group will be able to encourage the participation of others unless they themselves are active participants.

DEVELOPING AN INFORMATION BASE

The Lifegain committee needs solid factual information (1) to develop effective programs and provide accurate information about present health practices, problems, and concerns of the members of the community or organization, and (2) to make an assessment of the extent to which the organization's present health activities and personnel are currently meeting these needs.

The Lifegain health practices survey and the Lifegain norm indicator in Chapter 3 can be used as well as the Lifegain organizational support indicator which follows.

LIFEGAIN ORGANIZATIONAL SUPPORT INDICATOR

A number of key health practices that could be supported within an organization or community are listed below. Figure 2 concerns positive support for good health practices, Figure 3 analyzes negative forces that may need to be reduced. In each, choose the number that best indicates the level of support that now exists for these practices in your organization.

The data from the surveys you make can be fed back to the Lifegain task

FIGURE 2. Organizational Support Indicator.

How well is our organization or community doing in actively and consistently supporting people in their efforts to:	Very poorly	Poorly	Medium	Well	Very well
1. Engage in a regular, planned program of physical exercise?	1	2	3	4	5
2. Stop smoking?	1	2	3	4	5
3. Understand the significance of stress and what can be done to avoid its negative impact on personal health?	1	2	3	4	5
4. Achieve their correct weight and maintain it on a sustained basis?	1	2	3	4	5
5. Understand and follow sound nutritional practices, including eating a nutritional breakfast every day?	1	2	3	4	5
6. Avoid the overuse of caffeine, sugar, salt, and cholesterol producing foods?	1	2	3	4	5
7. Avoid the overuse and misuse of alcohol?	1	2	3	4	5
8. Avoid the overuse and misuse of drugs?	1	2	3	4	5
9. Have regular medical and dental examinations or health screenings and to follow up on the recommendations given?	1	2	3	4	5
10. Maintain their proper blood pressure?	1	2	3	4	5
11. Obtain sound health knowledge and maintain sound health practices?	1	2	3	4	5
12. Follow safety practices at home, at work, and on the highway?	1	2	3	4	5
13. Understand the importance of good mental health and deal effectively with mental health and emotional problems?	1	2	3	4	5
14. Develop and maintain positive human relations in their day-to-day activities?	1	2	3	4	5
15. Realize their full human potential?	1	2	3	4	5

FIGURE 3. Community Norm Indicator.

To what extent does your organization or community—	A great deal	Quite a lot	Some	Very little	Not at all
1. Consider health a low priority compared to other things?	1	2	3	4	5
2. Pay lip service to good health but not do much about it?	1	2	3	4	5
3. Place a low priority on funds for health education?	1	2	3	4	5
4. Criticize or put down people with a health problem (such as overweight or alcoholism), rather than giving them help?	1	2	3	4	5
5. Encourage people to eat more than they want or need?	1	2	3	4	5
6. Encourage people to drink more alcohol than is good for them?	1	2	3	4	5
7. Place a low emphasis on exercise?	1	2	3	4	5
8. Put people under unnecessary stress?	1	2	3	4	5
9. Indicate that smoking is OK by allowing smoking in general areas, by giving smoking related gifts?	1	2	3	4	5
10. Place a low priority on good safety practices?	1	2	3	4	5
11. Influence people to hold back expressing positive feelings about each other?	1	2	3	4	5
12. Place a low priority on life planning and fulfillment of individual potential?	1	2	3	4	5

forces and to the organization as a whole, to be used as the basis for program planning and individual goal setting.

If the results of your surveys are on the poor side, that will not be surprising. In the face of studies that show the high costs of poor health, remarkably few organizations are doing as much about health as one would expect, and almost none are doing as much as their individual members would like.

The charts below show some results from surveys taken in various companies that were examining their health practices and health cultures. They are shown here to indicate ways in which results can be presented, as well as to indicate the typically negative picture that is revealed before the change process begins.

Derived from the results of a health practices survey, Figure 4 shows the percentage of negative norms reported for each health area. Figure 5 gives a profile of a department's health norms and can be used for goal setting. Figure 6 summarizes one group's assessment of the organizational support it gets for good health practices.

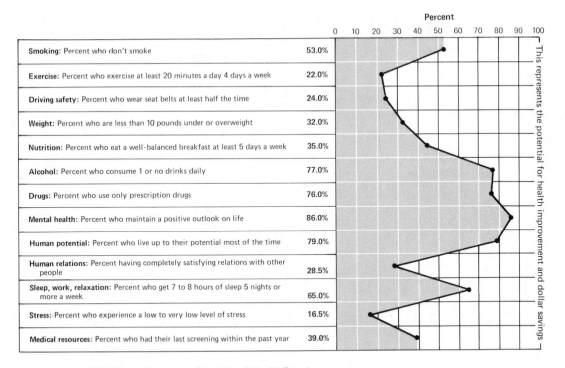

FIGURE 4. Summary of Individual Health Practices.

Some Other Sources of Information. Information can also be gathered by interviews, observations, and economic impact analysis. For example, a great deal can be learned by checking the food served and selected in the cafeteria; by noting smoking policies and patterns; by checking on the number of people making use of exercise facilities and practicing safety rules; by analyzing the number of accidents, the amount of absenteeism and its costs, the amount of money spent on hospitalization, and the amount spent on health education.

And it is important to find out what programs are already available and how much they are being used, so that you do not duplicate or compete with existing services but include them in an overall program.

Tasks of the Task Forces. Each task force has the responsibility to analyze data concerning its area of interest, to discover what is already being done in the organization or community in this area and what resources can be utilized inside and outside the organization, and to plan strategies for changing negative norms in that area.

As the task forces start to operate, many ideas will be suggested, usually

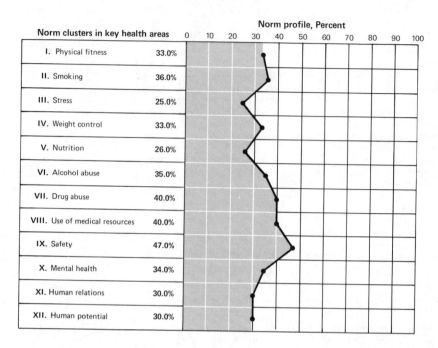

FIGURE 5.   The Lifeloss Norm Gap: Differences Between "What Is" and "What Could Be."

more than can be used. It's important to take time to be sure there is sound information on which to base any actions taken. Health is a complicated field, and a systematic analysis followed by a thoughtful setting of goals is the only way to assure ultimate success.

Phase II. Involvement

As soon as the tentative program is designed and the members of the leadership group are fully involved in their own change programs, the rest of the people in the organization are invited to participate in the introductory Lifegain workshops. In large organizations or communities, this can be carried out in phases, working with specific organizational units. A company might begin with the headquarters group or a specific factory unit. A community might begin with the city council, health department, or the leadership of the school system, volunteers and existing task forces and in setting up and conducting workshops.

The introductory workshop can last anywhere from two hours to several days, depending on its purpose and the extent of coverage that is desired. In most business organizations, a one-half to one-day workshop model has been found sufficient for introducing the program. The workshop is usually held

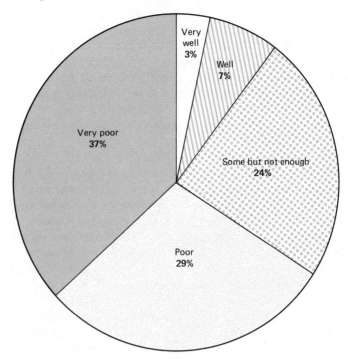

FIGURE 6. Organizational Support Indicator: Total of Responses to All Items.

during regular working hours; people have a choice of whether or not they wish to participate.

The workshop focuses on three concerns — understanding, identifying, and changing the culture. The first step, then, is to foster an understanding of the immense impact of the culture upon health practices, an awareness that these are choices, not requirements, and that we can do something about them. Usually this book can be used to help contribute to that understanding, and in the workshop, participants are encouraged to share their personal experiences and insights in relation to the various groups that they belong to.

The second step in the workshop is to identify where we are now, both as individuals and as part of an organization or a community, and where we want to be. The individual and group surveys will help identify these areas.

An individual might want to stop smoking, lose weight, or change some other health practice. The organization might wish to improve nutrition in its cafeteria and provide greater support for its exercise program. As these goals are set, it is important that a holistic health approach be taken, and that people realize how much working on one health practice can help another one.

The third step in the process is accomplishing change, and a number of alternatives are available to individual workshop participants. During the workshop, people learn what it takes to accomplish change and what possibilities are available to them.

Workshops need to be carefully planned. Audiovisuals and other materials are available, as well as suggested workshop agendas.

Phase III. Installing Change

Installing change is a multilevel process. The individual, the groups, the leadership, and the total organization must at one time or another be the focus of attention. People in the workshop have the opportunity to join task forces or Lifegain committees that have already been established, thus providing a new infusion of leadership and an opportunity for all participants to become personally involved in the leadership and the extension of the program. Individual self-help programs are available, as well as specialized groups dealing with particular problem areas, such as stress reduction or smoking cessation.

General Lifegain support groups are a key element of the change program. Through them people have an opportunity to gain support from one another in changing negative health practices and in maintaining the positive practices they have decided upon. They also have the chance, through discussions and exercises, to gain new information and skills that will be useful in improving their health and in assisting others to improve theirs.

The support group brings together people with a variety of concerns—one member might be primarily concerned with exercise, another with stress, and so on. The group situation makes it possible for people who are having trouble in one area to use their abilities to help people having trouble in another area. In the groups, people deal with their day to day problems, both individual and cultural.

The support group approach is primarily one of democratic, participatory decision making. Groups are essentially self-led, with specialists available at the beginning stages.

The support groups formed during the workshop consist of eight to 12 members who set as their goal the achievement of the individual goals of the members. The support groups meet regularly and their members are encouraged to be in contact with one another between meetings. Meetings provide an opportunity for the group members to report on how they are doing and to get the help and encouragement they might need for further improvements.

The support group also provides an opportunity for members to get new information by bringing in outside lecturers, films, etc.

While the individuals are working on their health practices, either on their own or more likely as members of the ongoing support group, organizational task forces work to create a positive environment supportive of what people are trying to accomplish. They might develop exercise facilities, encourage better nutrition in the food service, stress reduction programs — all as part of the total systematic change process.

In addition to working on their own change programs, each Lifegain participant is encouraged to participate in some type of outreach or task force activity. It has been found through experience that those people who work to bring the benefits of the program to others are much more likely to be able to hold on to the benefits that they have developed for themselves, and this is pointed out to all participants throughout the program. Outreach activities include the recruitment of new people for participation in the program, and the extension of the program to groups that have not had the opportunity to participate.

Task forces have the responsibility for tracking cultural change. They readminister norm instruments as needed, and present results so that members of the organization can follow the progress made.

One task force at a temple, for example, began to substitute fruits and nuts for the calorie laden sugary foods usually served following the Friday night service. It began by placing fruits and nuts on the table with the other food and found that more and more people were taking that choice.

Another task force arranged for the company cafeteria to stop featuring tempting pastries and to feature its nutritional salad bar instead.

Another task force readministered the Lifegain organizational support indicator after six months and presented the results on charts that were sent around for all support groups to see.

A company which had been characterized by its employees as a "stress factory" was convinced, after a task force study, that it would pay for them to examine and modify some of their current management practices and to provide opportunities for employees to participate in a stress reduction program to learn stress reducing techniques.

Supporting each other and working together for cultural change needs to become a way of life for an organization or community. It is through these individual and organizational changes that a positive health culture can be achieved. In Phase IV, efforts are made to sustain this achievement.

Phase IV. Sustaining Change

EVALUATION, RENEWAL, AND EXTENSION OF THE PROGRAM

How well are you doing? Check it out with evaluations at strategic times in task force meetings.

Have a full-scale evaluation at least once a year. It adds motivation. When people know someone is going to ask for a report on what they're doing, they're more apt to get it done. It is important to remember that evaluations should cover cultural change as well as individual achievements.

What can you use to evaluate? You can use the same instruments that you used for the initial surveys, simply repeating them to see how far the group has come. Large corporations can also have an economic impact task force

conduct an annual review to see what improvements have occurred in insurance costs, absenteeism, illness, and other factors that affect productivity
and cost effectiveness.

A small group can combine the evaluation and discussion with a trip to the
beach or a mountain resort for a weekend.

A community group of former migrants who used the system, renews and
evaluates its efforts through ongoing committees responsible for health care,
child development, and community services. In addition, once a year a comprehensive evaluation meeting is held at which the consultants come back to
be part of the assessment.

Evaluations such as these can be used to encourage the continued renewal
and extension of the program. Most organizations also form alumni groups
that bring new health programs and new ideas on a continuing basis.

And just as the individual Lifegain programs include reaching out to others,
Lifegain organization programs tend to extend beyond the borders of the
organization. A business organization finds it is extending the program to
families and community leaders; a community finds that others outside its
borders get involved. People involved in Lifegain find that its principles and
the change process they have learned are valuable for other problems with
which they are confronted.

THE TEN COMMANDMENTS OF ORGANIZATION AND COMMUNITY CHANGE

Programs necessarily take on their own unique qualities, and there are no
rules comparable in status to a general commandment. (In fact, most rules
have to be tempered as they are implemented on a day to day basis.) However, there are a few rules that come close to being necessary for a successful
change program. Since they are valid both for individuals and groups, they
bear repeating here, though you have become familiar with them in principle
throughout our discussions of the Lifegain process.

> Personal *Involvement* vs. leaving it to others
> *Caring* for Each Other vs. being exclusively concerned about ourselves
> *Health Emphasis* vs. illness emphasis
> Based on *Sound Data* vs. hunches and wishful thinking
> Freedom of *Choice* vs. telling others what to do
> Measurable *Results* vs. focus on activities
> Sustained *Achievement* vs. campaign-type efforts
> *Systematic Approaches* vs. piecemeal solutions
> Positive *Support* vs. negative blame placing
> *Fun* and *Pleasure Orientation* vs. grim scare tactics

You might ask yourself the following questions periodically in your program to make sure you are still following these principles.

Does your program focus on cultural change?
Does it help develop the internal capabilities of the people in the organization rather than relying solely on outside consultants?

Does your program provide personal involvement of the people rather than leaving leadership to a few?

Is your program based on sound data rather than on hunches or wishful thinking?

Does your program provide for freedom of choice rather than telling others what to do?

Does your program focus on obtaining specific goals and measurable results rather than focusing on keeping-busy activities?

Does your program emphasize steady, sustained, long-term efforts rather than short-term campaigns?

Does your program have a well-planned, systematic approach rather than offering uncoordinated piecemeal solutions?

Does your program look toward solving problems and giving positive support rather than negative blame placing?

Does your program encourage caring for each other?

Does your program have a wellness rather than an illness emphasis?

Is your program fun?

LIFEGAIN IS FOR EVERYONE

As you work together with others on your Lifegain program don't leave anyone out who would like to be included. Sick people, for example, can often be the "healthiest" people of all when it comes to caring for others. One woman who was in the terminal stages of cancer when she first became involved in the Lifegain program, became one of the most committed and contributing members of her group. She recognized that living fully was even more important than living long and inspired others because of her courage and commitment. Another member was confined to a wheel chair for life because of a childhood accident but saw no reason to restrict her life or her health supporting activities because of it.

Older people also make excellent Lifegain group members. They often have maturity, energy, and time to contribute, all of which can mean a great deal to the success of the Lifegain program. Nor does Lifegain have to be a luxury program for the well-to-do. All people have much to gain and much to contribute. When members are welcomed as a part of the overall program, they can serve to enrich not only their own lives but also the lives of the other members.

One Lifegain group that went out of its way to see that its members were representative of all segments of the community found that its members could not only work together on the more traditional "health" problems but could also work successfully on some of the more difficult community problems that were getting in the way of healthier lifestyles.

HAVING FUN WHILE YOU'RE BRINGING ABOUT CHANGE

Working on a Lifegain program can and should be fun. It should not be just another chore added to the stress that too many of us already feel in our lives. When we are working at cultural change, it is long-range change that we are trying to bring about. If it's not fun, we won't keep at it long enough for it to make any difference.

Your own joy at a new relationship, new exercise patterns, new nutrition programs, and most importantly, new ways of reaching out to others will in the long run make all the difference.

Many people have found some of their best friends in this way.

Some people have even found themselves.

CONCLUSION: CONTINUING YOUR LIFEGAIN PROGRAM FOR A LIFETIME

Whether you continue the Lifegain program in formal meetings with others or simply go on your own, you need to keep your efforts recharged. You don't want to slip back to the negative ways. Don Ardell, the author of an outstanding book on wellness, makes our options very clear when he suggests that "high level wellness," as much trouble as it might be to secure, is infinitely better than the "low level worseness" that we have become accustomed to in our society.

You want total, permanent, sustained change, a superhealth of feeling better and enjoying yourself to the maximum for the rest of your life. This involves continually being alert to old or new culture traps, remembering how they work and how you can combat them so you can constantly be in charge of your own health and life.

In both your organizations and in your own life, you can take part in the idea whose time has come: the creative use of cultural influences to help people achieve high level wellness.

People sometimes ask what the essential differences are between the Lifegain approach and other approaches to health change. We believe that these essential differences are freedom, cultural support, and caring. Freedom in the sense that we are no longer blocked by the culture that surrounds us; cultural support in the sense that we focus not only on ourselves but also on the environment in which we live; and caring in the sense that we care not only about ourselves but about each other.

Lifegain is a forward step in the evolution of health practices, and you are part of it. The focus on health cultures — the crux of the Lifegain program — means a new dimension for you. You can see now how the cultural focus enhances your importance as an individual, giving you the kind of support you need to develop and sustain the best that is possible for you.

And it gives you freedom. Instead of being a victim of what happens to you, you are learning to control your own life. You are involved in what happens to your own health and future and the health and future of your family and friends as well. You are in charge, in a new and exciting way, of being responsible for your own life and supporting other people in taking responsibility for theirs.

It can be the most important step you have ever taken in your evolution toward better health. And if the system spreads, as it looks like it will, many people will be able to strive successfully for better health, rooting out poor health before it develops and making it possible to achieve high level wellness both as individuals and as societies

Most of the individual efforts in the world are going to come to naught if they aren't supported by the culture. Only a few people are going to jog if there are not other joggers; few people are going to be the only salad eaters in town; few people want to be the only thin person in a world of fat people. Most of us need the social support from the people around us in our homes and work places.

A few people may have the willpower to change despite massive cultural obstacles, but most of us find such change extremely difficult. To go it alone requires the stamina of a hero. We admire heroes, but wouldn't it be better to live in a world where they were not necessary? To paraphrase Plato, "A society is in jeopardy when a person has to be a hero to do the right thing." The cultural approach of Lifegain can help us create worlds where "the right thing" is the norm. Instead of asking people to change their behavior and then making it almost impossible for them to do it in the environmental framework provided them, we can now work together to provide the environment in which most people will succeed.

We offer the Lifegain program as a systematic, workable way to help people build the kind of supportive cultures that they need for their own personal well-being.

Miraculous things can happen, more quickly and more widely than you might think possible, if people get cultural support. Not only can they reach better health, but they can also work together in a non blame-placing way, feel more free to make suggestions, listen more actively to others, look for culture traps in other areas, and search for better ways to make things work better for everyone.

This focus on changing the health culture—the crux of the Lifegain program—means a new dimension for you and others in your strivings for better health, going deeper, rooting out poor health before it develops, and making it possible for them to achieve high-level wellness both as individuals and as societies. It can be the most important step you have ever taken in your personal progress toward superhealth and to the fuller use of your human potential.

Total wellness is not a fantasy. It is a reality you can achieve. Total wellness involves *you* plus you-and-your-culture, practicing a lifestyle that can bring you and those you care for the sustained total health that should be the birthright of our and future generations.

We wish you good luck with your Lifegain program for yourself and with your Lifegain system for your organization, community, or family. Enjoy superhealth and enjoy the process of getting there.

Materials for setting up your own Lifegain workshops or for planning change programs in organizations can be obtained at nominal cost from: Human Resources Institute (HRI), Tempe Wick Road, Morristown, NJ 07960.

A Brief Annotated Bibliography

Allen, Robert F., with Charlotte Kraft. *Beat The System.* New York: Mc-Graw-Hill, 1980.

The concepts and methods of Normative Systems, the cultural change process upon which Lifegain is based, are described with illustrations from its application to a variety of cultures.

Allen, Robert F. with C. Kraft, et al. *Normative Systems Management: A Handbook for the Analysis of Cultures and the Planning of Change by Groups, Organizations, and Communities.* Morristown, N.J.: HRI Press, 1978.

Provides a step by step process for planning successful change programs based on the Normative Systems change model. Provides specific illustrations drawn from actual change experiences in a variety of areas.

Ardell, Donald B. *High Level Wellness: An Alternative to Doctors, Drugs, and Disease.* Emmaus, Pa.: Rodale Press, 1977.

A bright and lively guidebook with practical suggestions for achieving high level wellness. Ardell emphasizes nutritional awareness, stress management, physical fitness, and environmental sensitivity for the individual, but also discusses ways to create new and better health planning systems for all of us.

Benson, Herbert, M.D. *The Relaxation Response.* New York: Avon, 1975.

A synthesis of literature and information regarding meditative techniques, plus a method to help us deal with the increased stress of contemporary life. Dr. Benson deals with the physiological aspects of stress and its relation to hypertension, as well as the religious and spiritual discoveries about relaxation through the ages.

Carlson, Richard. *The End of Medicine.* New York: Wiley, 1975.

A penetrating analysis of some of the most crucial myths and destructive aspects of our medical and illness orientation, with thoughtful suggestions on making use of medical expertise within the larger framework of a health oriented society.

Cooper, Kenneth, H., M.D. *Aerobics.* New York: Bantam Books, 1968.

Contains a simple, easy to follow guide to one of the world's most popular and widely accepted fitness programs. Cooper uses normal activity to improve overall health and offers charts, tables, and, most importantly, his special point system, which helps you in planning a program for yourself and for measuring the results.

Dubin, Harry; Liss, Moe; and Raynor, Doug. *Coping Successfully.* New York: Irvington Press, 1980.

A how-to manual to implement successful change in various organizational and community settings. Blends theory with practical applications.

Ferguson, Tom, M.D. *Medical Self Care: Access to Self Help Tools.* New York: Simon and Schuster, 1980.

This carefully edited collection of pieces from one of the nation's leading self-help journals can help you approach your own self-help care with confidence.

246

Fixx, James F., *The Complete Book of Running*. New York: Random House, 1977.

Fixx's book covers every aspect of running, including the "why," the "how," and the controversies. It is a virtual encyclopedia on the subject and is readable, well-structured, and informative. It is especially good for the novice but carries material for runners of any level.

Gallwey, Timothy. *Inner Tennis*. New York: Random House, 1976.

Although focused on tennis, this is more than a book about the one sport. There are valuable insights on ways to tune in to our bodies, nonjudgmental attitudes toward our exercise efforts, and guides to using imagery and modeling that can affect many aspects of our lives.

Glasser, William, M.D. *Positive Addiction*. New York: Harper and Row, 1976.

A book about the kind of behavior that can strengthen us and help us fulfill our potential for high level wellness. Glasser offers some important concepts concerning the psychology of personal behavior and a program for developing positive addictions as a substitute for destructive addictions and unhealthy lifestyles.

Harris, Sara, and Allen, Robert F. *The Quiet Revolution*. New York: Rawson Associates, 1978.

A true story of a successful change program based on a Normative Systems-Lifegain change model. In this program, migrant workers successfully transformed their human environments, their company, and themselves. This book tells how this was accomplished from the perspective of both the workers and the company that employed them.

James, Muriel, and Jongeward, Dorothy. *Born To Win*. Menlo Park, Ca.: Addison-Wesley, 1971.

The authors interpret transactional analysis (TA) and Gestalt oriented concepts and provide a multitude of do-it-yourself exercises to help develop increased self-awareness. These enable you to analyze your interrelationships with others and do something about changing them if you want to.

Linde, Shirley. *The Whole Health Catalogue*. New York: Rawson Associates, 1977.

A catalog chock full of information on diet, exercise, energy, sex, sleep, increasing the quantity and quality of life, and many more aspects of the health world. There are tests you can do yourself, directories of health services, and practical information on where to go and how to send for what you need.

Maslow, Abraham. *Toward a Psychology of Being*. New York: Van Nostrand, 1968.

Maslow, a learned authority on motivation and personality, explains his theories on self-actualization, peak experiences, creativity, and personal growth. A valuable resource for people wishing to work on making use of their full potential.

Mayer, Jean, M.D. *A Diet for Living*. New York: David McKay, 1975.

An accepted authority on nutrition gives facts on nutrients, obesity, diet, etc., cutting through many of the fallacies. In readable question and answer forms and handy charts, Mayer gives us much information and many practical suggestions on the choosing and preparation of foods.

Montague, Ashley. *Touching: The Human Significance of Skin*. New York: Harper and Row, 1971.

The renowned anthropologist analyzes the skin as the prime organ of relation to the outside world. He examines the cultural influences and implications and sug-

gests a return to more primitive interactions as a defense against the dehumaniza-
tion of our increasingly technological society.

Peele, Stanton. *Love and Addiction.* New York: Signet, 1975.

An insightful look at the relationship between various forms of addiction in our
society. It can help people to consider their own addictions and to substitute more
positive forms of behavior.

Robbins, Lewis C., M.D., and Hall, Jack, M.D. *How to Practice Prospective
Medicine.* Indianapolis: Slaymaker Enterprises, 1970.

An instructional handbook designed for medical practitioners describing the development of prospective medicine and the method of health hazard appraisal. More
specifically, it explains the use of the *Giller-Gesner Risk Manual,* the core ingredient
of prospective medicine.

Selye, Hans, M.D. *Stress Without Distress.* New York: Signet, 1974.

An enlightening overview of the nature of stress and distress and its relationship to
work and leisure goals. Includes a method for the constructive management of
stress and a philosophical framework to help you examine and shape some basic
life decisions.

U.S. Congress, Senate, Select Committee on Nutrition and Human Needs.
Dietary Goals for the United States, Second Edition. U.S. Government
Printing Office: Washington, D.C., December 1977.

A detailed report of the Senate committee's findings on United States dietary
needs, with discussions of the research findings and the pros and cons that led to
each goal. While this is heavy going in spots, filled with statistics and tables, it is
valuable for its background information and its recommendations. This is the revised version.

Vickery, Donald M., M.D., and Fries, James F., M.D. *Take Care of Yourself:
A Consumer's Guide to Medical Care.* Reading, Ma.: Addison-Wesley,
1977.

A do-it-yourself guide to medical care sponsored by Blue Cross/Blue Shield that is
full of information to help you make sound medical decisions for yourself and your
family. It covers home treatment and what to expect of the doctor for 70 of the
most common complaints. It gives help on choosing the right doctor and the right
medical facility and is designed to help you save time and money by handling many
ailments yourself.